"THIS BOOK COULD SAVE YOUR LIFE."

"By reading and following the suggestions you can reduce your chances of developing the 'common' diseases of aging and live to your maximum lifespan. The dietary changes outlined will reduce your risk of developing heart disease, cancer, diabetes, arthritis, impotence, senility, and serious digestive disorders.

"We all must age. The trick is to live to our maximum lifespan without succumbing to any of the typical diseases normally thought to be part of 'getting old.'

"You *are* what you eat, and we can slowly undo a lifetime of mistaken notions about your ability to eat as you will using the 'cubes' I have devised at the end of each chapter. Patiently and slowly you will notice changes. There are no *instant* methods for reversing a lifetime of faulty eating and drinking patterns. But, by incorporating the changes I call for in this book you will notice an increase in energy and less fatigue in the afternoon or early evening. Your bowel problems will likely disappear while your skin, hair, and nails will maintain or regain their luster. Your interest in and performance of the sexual pleasures will also improve, so long as you continue to follow the dietary changes I have outlined for you."

—from the Preface

BEVERLY HILLS DIET LIFETIME PLAN by Judy Mazel
BEVERLY HILLS MEDICAL DIET by Judy Mazel
THE BRAND NAME NUTRITION COUNTER by Jean Carper
COMPLETE BOOK OF HOMEOPATHY by Michael Weiner, Ph.D.
   and Kathleen Goss
COMPLETE SCARSDALE MEDICAL DIET by Herman Tarnower
   and Samm Sinclair Baker
DIET FOR LIFE by Francine Price
E: THE ESSENTIAL VITAMIN by Herbert Bailey
EARL MINDELL'S VITAMIN BIBLE FOR YOUR KIDS
   by Earl Mindell
EATING FOR TWO: THE COMPLETE PREGNANCY NUTRITION
   COOKBOOK by Isaac Cronin & Gail Sforza Brewer
FOOD ADDITIVES BOOK by Nicholas Freydberg, Ph.D. and
   Willis A. Gortner, Ph.D.
GH3-WILL IT KEEP YOU YOUNG LONGER? by Herbert Bailey
GIFT OF HEALTH by Richard Shames, M.D. and
   Karilee Halo Shames, R.N., Ph.D.
HEALTH FOR THE WHOLE PERSON by Arthur C. Hastings, Ph.D.,
   ed., James Fadiman, Ph.D. and James S. Gordon, M.D.
HERB BOOK by John Lust
HOW TO LIVE 365 DAYS A YEAR THE SALT FREE WAY
   by J. Peter Bruns, Dorothy Love, and Dr. Asa Weinberg
JANE BRODY'S NUTRITION BOOK by Jane Brody
NATURAL FOODS CALORIE COUNTER by Carl Lissance,
   Mele Olsen, and Phil Groves
NUTRITION AND VITAMIN THERAPY by Dr. Michael Lesser
NUTRITION AGAINST AGING by Michael Weiner
PSYCHODIETETICS by Dr. E. Choraskin and Dr. W. M. Ringsdorf
   with Arline Brecher
PRITIKIN PERMANENT WEIGHT LOSS MANUAL
   by Nathan Pritikin
PRITIKIN PROGRAM FOR DIET & EXERCISE by Nathan Pritikin
   with Patrick McGrady
SECRETS OF LIFE EXTENSION by John A. Mann
SPIRULINA by Larry Switzer
WHICH VITAMINS DO YOU NEED? by Martin Ebon

NUTRITION AGAINST AGING

**Michael A. Weiner Ph.D.
and
Kathleen Goss**

BANTAM BOOKS
TORONTO · NEW YORK · LONDON · SYDNEY

This book is not intended to replace
your own physician with whom you should
consult before taking any medication or
considering treatment.

NUTRITION AGAINST AGING

A Bantam Book / November 1983

Reproductions by Robert J. Sabuda.

*Permission granted by the American Heart Association to reprint
tables from ''Coronary Heart Disease'' by Robert Levy, 1981
from* Arteriosclerosis Vol. 1 #5.

ISBN 0-553-23642-3

Published simultaneously in the United States and Canada

PRINTED IN THE UNITED STATES OF AMERICA

H   0 9 8 7 6 5 4 3 2 1

CONTENTS

FOREWORD

An Ounce of Prevention Is Worth a Pound of Inheritance!

My father and his father both died too young from heart attacks. I was thrown into a panic while still in college, rushing back and forth between the oxygen tent and my biology classes.

Soon after my father "recovered" from his first heart attack I failed my only college course—genetics! How could I believe that genes, not environment, controlled our destiny, with so poor a health gene pool in my family?

As my studies developed—first in cell biology, later in human nutrition, medical anthropology, and epidemiology—it became clear to me that our environment *does*, in fact, shape our health. In different regions of the world, I noticed that certain *nations* seemed to "die" from "their" diseases while other nations were somewhat "immune." My father, may he rest in peace, died not from a heart attack but from malnutrition which gradually brought about the ultimate end. Likewise with the other 650,000(!) people in the United States who died from coronary heart disease (in 1978). Virtually *all of these deaths* were the product of the chief disease of aging, and preventable through exercise, nutrition, and vitamin and mineral supplements.

Cancer will kill nearly 400,000 people this year—the result of genes inherited from a parent or grandparent who died from this agonizing killer illness, or a product of environmental stresses which can be controlled. The leading experts in cancer themselves now agree that cancer is basically a preventable disease, that it is *not* of mysterious origins. We know for example that workers in certain industries—rubber, polyvinyl chloride, creosote, and asbestos—all die much more frequently from this illness than the general population. Looking around the world, other patterns have emerged. Even relatively primitive people associate many diseases with living habits, including food. All major religions have food prohibitions, and in the case of the Seventh-day Adventists, who abstain from tobacco, alcohol, and meat, the followers are rewarded with a much *lower* rate of many forms of cancer.

As my studies intensified in the area of nutrition, I grew even *more* certain that our basic genetic inheritance was significantly aided by rational principles of living— that is, what we eat and drink (or do *not* eat and drink!) played a *key role* in preventing or speeding up the principal diseases of our middle and later years.

The old "nature versus nurture" controversy, I had decided back at Queens College, was probably resolved on the side of nurture (I subsequently received an *F* in the course from my genetics teacher, who sat on the opposite side of the dispute). That viewpoint now seems to have the blessings of the most respected scientists in medical research, at least for now, in the heart disease, cancer, and diabetes arenas of study.

The other *diseases* of *aging* treated here, by myself and my coauthor Kathleen Goss, are *also* largely *preventable*, and it is only a matter of time before the medical community agrees, and acts to instruct their patients in the ways of preventive nutrition, as outlined here.

But for these changes to occur the medical community must eventually overcome its mental barrier. All of modern science has, for the past century at least, viewed disease as resulting from "the intrusion of some positive factor, some *res morbi*, be it a parasite or poison" (Hopkins, in Guggenheim 1979).

Yet, as we will show in this book, the principal diseases of aging are primarily the result of a *minus;* that is, due to *dietary deficiencies*. And, the diseases we have come to dread are largely *preventable* or partially controlled through diet and nutrient supplements.

How to Use this Book

But merely telling you that these diseases are preventable through diet, without showing you *how* to make the necessary changes, simply and gradually, would be a useless academic discourse. To better serve this need we have created a series of nine "building blocks of health." Each chapter concludes with a block containing nine sections. In each block are ranked protective factors relating to the cause, prevention, or reversal of the illness of aging discussed in that chapter. Relative "weights" are given to each factor and a "score" is calculated for each preventable illness. Thus, by calculating the score you earn at the end of each chapter and then by adding up the totals, you can see how close you are to achieving the ideal overall protective health rating of 486 points.

We suggest that you score your "aging profile" just as soon as you've read each chapter. Then a "tally card" is used, on page 00, to enable you to *rate yourself* and see how far you have to go to score an *A* in the aging game!

At three-month intervals you can use these handy blocks to see how many more points you've scored against disease, aging, and in positive beauty gain. Then, by again adding your totals you will be able to rate your progress. In this way you can slowly improve your "inner environment" and calculate just how far you've gone in building a solid pattern of healthful aging. For the first time a quantitative method is yours to use in the puzzle of successful aging.

Keep in mind that no program for health should be undertaken without medical supervision. Certain vitamins can be toxic at high levels, so your doctor's guidance is essential.

MICHAEL WEINER

PREFACE

This book could save your life. By reading and following the suggestions you can reduce your chances of developing the "common" diseases of aging and live to your maximum lifespan. The dietary changes outlined herein will reduce your risk of developing heart disease, cancer, diabetes, arthritis, impotence, senility, and serious digestive disorders. These are no longer the diseases of mysterious origin they once were.

By penetrating the conspiracy of confusion I am now able to demonstrate the dietary links in the chain of disease development and explain how simple shifts in relative food *portions*, foods you *now eat*, can be accomplished to keep you healthier longer, or reverse gradually, the diseases associated with aging.

Defeatists say, "Why bother with nutrition? When it's your turn to go, you go," and they continue to smoke, drink, eat endless quantities of refined foods, heavy fats, salt, and sugar, and generally act as though nothing has been learned in the past ten years. The facts though, weigh heavily against this kind of falsely "fatalistic" posture. We now know that we can live to our maximum life span without succumbing to any of the typical diseases normally thought to be part of "getting old." To convince my patients of this I ask them, "Tell me, don't you think that some of the food you eat can end your life right now?"

Then, after explaining how an overdose of common table salt or caffeine or even sugar, in susceptible individuals, could end their existence, I go on to show how gradually we, in fact, hasten our own demise by pretending not to know what effects nutrition or the lack thereof, has on the disease process.

Although we all must age, age does not mean sickness! Many people simply live to a ripe old age and gradually weaken, as their metabolic "machinery" runs out of energy (that is, their DNA codes their cells to age). They do not become a burden to themselves or to others. Now we all know someone who is 90 years old and still drinking two glasses of whisky each and every day *or* smoking two packs of cigarettes a day and eating white bread and ice cream as their staple foods! I call these types nutritional rogues. They are *not* the model for those of us blessed with less vigorous constitutions. Further, I have long believed that even the old rogue who abused all health rules and lived to 96 could have lived to the age of Moses (120), had he or she followed the simple dietary plans outlined in this book.

You *are* what you eat and you can slowly undo a lifetime of mistaken notions about your ability to eat as you will using the "cubes" I have devised at the end of each chapter. Patiently and slowly you will notice changes. There are no *instant* methods for reversing a lifetime of faulty eating and drinking patterns. Let anyone who promises otherwise prove it with reams of statistically valid data. But, by incorporating the changes I call for in this book you will notice an increase in energy and less fatigue in the afternoon or early evening. Your bowel problems will likely disappear while your skin, hair, and nails will maintain or regain their luster. Your interest in, and performance of, the sexual pleasures will also improve, so long as you continue to follow the dietary changes I have outlined for you.

These are the *outward* signs that you are gaining on the aging process and are physical manifestations that *internally* you are winning the battle against premature disease and aging.

If you are skeptical about these claims, why not compare the suggestions I make in the following pages with your own ideas about nutrition? You will quickly see that I do not dictate an ideal diet, but that I *encourage* you in your idiosyncratic and ethnic preferences. By learning to slowly alter your food choices you will feel better and begin to *worry* less about diet and health. This easy to follow program of dietary changes will take the guesswork out of nutrition while allowing you to enjoy your middle and older years, and to devote more time to worthier causes than your own digestive tract!

To see just how serious I am and how solid my references are, please read the chapter which discusses the disease you fear most. Then, move on to another chapter of interest. In a few months you will be on the road to a worry-free nutritional plan for maximum longevity.

NUTRITION AGAINST AGING

1

DON'T LOSE HEART!

The Heart Disease Riddle Unraveled

There Goes My Heart . . . or, Need it Go?

Science, like religion, can only suggest a set of coordinates for us to follow. Absolute rules of conduct do not apply to all people in the same way. Killing, for example, may be exonerated or even condoned during times of war, even by religious leaders. To present a set of dietary guidelines which will work to prevent atherosclerosis ("hardening of the arteries") for *all* people, would be a medical dream. Unfortunately, such hard and fast rules do not apply to *all* people.

To prevent heart disease, ethnic, idiosyncratic, and other differences between people would have some of us requiring very low saturated fat, high-fiber diets with ample intake of vitamins B_6, C, E, and the minerals magnesium and zinc. Those of us not hereditarily prone to coronary heart disease (CHD) could very likely eat with a great degree of freedom, avoiding some or all of these nutritional coordinates, and avoid the disease of the century just as well. However, if you are reading this chapter you probably have a family history of CHD or fear you are too inactive, and would like to do what you can to lessen your "risk factors." A key point to remember is that CHD is *not* a "natural process of aging" (Levy 1981), and that we *can* reduce our risk by focusing on prevention, mainly through exercise and *easy* dietary changes, as you will see.

America's Number One Killer

Of all the diseases which haunt the American consciousness and drive us to consume unparalleled quantities of remedies, preventives, and medical care, we have most reason to fear coronary heart disease, for it is by far the leading cause of death in the United States, and it strikes most cruelly, the middle-aged or older individuals. In 1978, 650,000 people in the United States died from coronary heart disease; 150,000 of those people were over 65. By contrast, 400,000 died of cancer. Even among younger people coronary heart disease is a fearsome killer, responsible for almost a third of all deaths in people from 35 to 64. When we add to coronary heart disease the other cardiovascular diseases, most notably strokes, the figures are truly staggering: nearly a million deaths a year owing to the deterioration of the cardiovascular system.

The cost to the American public of CHD can be measured in terms of dollars as well as lives. At least $27 billion is drained from our resources each year by this disease—$6 billion in direct medical costs, and upward of $20 billion in lost productivity (Levy 1981, p. 312).

Perhaps the most astonishing fact about coronary heart disease, is that at the beginning of this century it was relatively unknown as a cause of death. Myocardial infarction, or heart attacks, appeared infrequently in the medical literature of the day. Yet by 1940, CHD had become the leading cause of death in the United States as well as in several other countries!

We now know that coronary heart disease has been with us throughout history. It has even been identified in Egyptian mummies 2,000 years old. But the underlying condition that leads to CHD, known as atherogenesis, may go on for years without being manifested in observable symptoms such as heart attacks, chest pain, or sudden death.

Atherosclerosis: the silent killer. Atherosclerosis begins with the deposition of fat, particularly cholesterol ester, on the inner layers of the large arteries. The reason why this occurs is not entirely known, but it may be a response to injury, blood flow, chronic irritation, or other factors. Cells on the inner lining of the artery proliferate at the same time, so that eventually these fats and cells, along with fibrous tissue and crystals from the cholesterol, begin to form scars and plaques. While this process may begin early in life—perhaps as early as the teens—it can go unrecognized for years. It's only when the plaques become so dense that they interfere with blood flow, or when a piece of plaque breaks away to obstruct a blood vessel elsewhere, or when a blood clot forms on the surface of the artery wall, that such observable and often life-threatening symptoms as anginal pain or heart attacks occur.

We might speculate that earlier in history when the average life expectancy was considerably shorter than it is today, and the accumulated damage to the heart would not be great enough to be fatal, such symptoms might have been less likely to occur. Even so, there have always been at least a few older people in every society, and so we must ask why the death rate for coronary heart disease has skyrocketed in the twentieth century, until recently when a *downward* trend has been recorded.

There seems to be little doubt that life-style-related factors, including the decline in daily physical activity and the change in the Western diet, are significant contributory factors.

The mystery of the declining death rate. But if we look at the statistics more closely, we will see perhaps even more compelling evidence that life-style factors—factors under our control—are directly related to the incidence of fatal heart attacks. If you look at Table 1.1, you will see that after rising steadily during this century, the death rate for coronary heart disease slowed in the late 1950s, and then sometime during the 1960s began to decline. The decline began first among nonwhites and females, and later among white males. It began first in the Western states and continues to be more marked there. (New Mexico and Hawaii have the lowest rates, perhaps because of their large Latino and Asian populations, whose diets may contain more protective nutrients and fewer "danger foods," as discussed later in this chapter.) Nationwide, the coronary heart disease death rate has declined by about 23 percent from 1969 to 1977 for all segments of the population, despite regional, sex, and racial differences. Accompanying this drop in death rate, there is some preliminary evidence from autopsies of men who died of noncoronary causes—such as accidents, violence, or natural causes—that the rate of atherosclerosis also may have slowed (Levy 1981, p. 315). Moreover, death rates for other atherosclerotic diseases, particularly strokes, have also declined. In fact, the decline in the death rates from strokes has been even greater than that from CHD. So significant has been the decline in the death rate from cardiovascular diseases, that there has been a concomitant, measurable *increase* in life expectancy of over two years during the last decade.

Table 1.1

U.S. Death Rates for Coronary Artery Disease,
1940–1978

Year	Death rate*
1940	207.2
1945	208.2
1950	226.4
1955	226.0
1960	238.5
1965	237.7
1970	228.1
1975	196.1
1978	180.9

* Rate per 100,000 population; age adjusted to the U.S. population, 1940.

Source: National Center for Health Statistics

(From Levy 1981, p. 313)

Table 1.2

*Trends in the Death Rate for Coronary Heart Disease
Among Men Aged 35–74 Years in Selected Countries
1969 and 1977*

Country	Change in rate (%)	Rate per 100,000 population*	
		1969	1977
United States	−22.6	864.7	669.6
Australia	−19.0	843.7	683.1
Japan	−18.8	126.3	102.6†
Canada	−11.3	703.3	624.1
Israel	−11.1	653.3	581.0‡
Norway	−7.9	583.0	537.1
Belgium	−4.3	446.1	426.8‡
New Zealand	−3.4	773.4	747.1
Finland	−1.7	893.7	878.1‡
Italy	−1.1	313.0	309.6§
Scotland	−0.6	813.8	808.6
Czechoslovakia	+0.4	587.9	590.4§
England and Wales	+1.4	662.1	671.7
Denmark	+1.8	566.1	576.3
Ireland	+2.3	662.2	677.7§
Netherlands	+4.6	478.7	500.5
France	+6.0	195.2	207.0‡
Austria	+6.3	428.3	455.3
Sweden	+6.9	524.0	560.1
West Germany	+7.2	427.3	458.1
Switzerland	+7.6	290.4	312.7
Northern Ireland	+10.8	782.4	867.1
Hungary	+13.0	441.6	499.2
Yugoslavia	+23.0	185.0	227.6
Romania	+39.2	170.5	237.4
Bulgaria	+41.4	299.4	423.5
Poland	+65.0	186.5	307.8

*Age-averaged.

†Already very low, the death rate from heart disease in Japan dropped even further between 1969 and 1977. The figure is thought to be so low owing to the fish, vegetables, and dietary rice staples and cultural factors which emphasize cooperative behavior.

‡1976.

§1975.

Source: Unpublished data provided by Dr. F. H. Epstein and Dr. Z. Pisa. (From Levy p. 317)

Figure 1.1

*Death Rates for Coronary Heart Disease by Country:
Men 35–74 Years of Age**

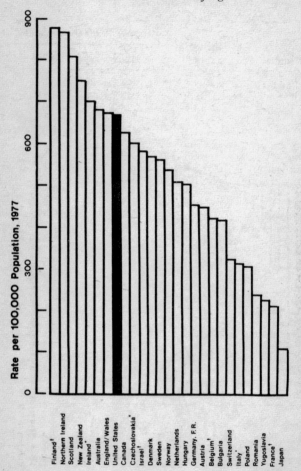

*1975 data.
†1976 data.

Source: Prepared by NHLBI; data from the World Health Organization.
(From Levy p. 318)

Figure 1.1 (cont.)

Death Rates for Coronary Heart Disease by Country:
Men 35–74 Years of Age

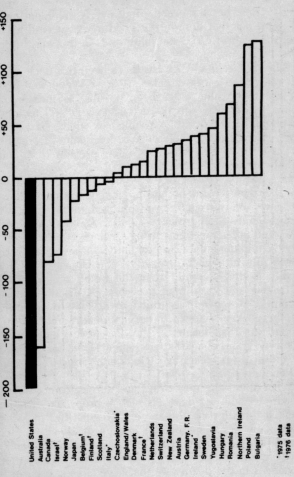

* 1975 data
† 1976 data

Source: Prepared by NHLBI; data from the World Health Organization

(From Levy, p. 318)

Nor has this decline in the CHD death rate been restricted to the United States. In Table 1.2 you will see that the trend has occurred in other industrialized countries as well. The decline has been the greatest in the United States; but lest we become overly confident, we must point out that despite this good news, we still have one of the highest CHD mortality rates in the world (see Figure 1.1).

Why the decline? Why has there been this decline in death rates from cardiovascular diseases? We should first point out that while it has been possible to measure a decline in mortality, this doesn't necessarily tell us anything about CHD morbidity. People may still be having as many heart attacks as before. We don't know from the statistics if the disease is actually being prevented, or if it is only being treated more effectively.

One possible reason for the decline in mortality, then, might be that treatment has improved. Coronary care units now take an aggressive approach in treating the myocardial infarction patient—monitoring heart rate and rhythm and other functions, using cardiopulmonary resuscitative equipment and surgical interventions that were not available in earlier times. But the change in CHD mortality is much greater than the number of patients hospitalized—successfully or not—in specialized coronary care units. Moreover, according to at least one study, while there are now fewer in-hospital deaths among coronary patients than formerly, the one-, two-, and three-year survival rates of heart attack patients have not changed from those of ten years ago (Goldberg, Szklo, Tonascia, and Kennedy 1979).

What about the new drugs and surgical procedures? Beta-adrenergic-blocking drugs such as propanolol may be helping to prevent life-threatening irregularities in heart rhythm. Other calcium-channel antagonists are also under investigation for possible treatment of cardiac patients. Such drugs offer hope for the future, but don't account for the changes in the death rate that have already occurred. Coronary artery bypass surgery, which has become a somewhat common medical procedure in recent years, does *not* seem to be contributing to a decline in the death rate, although it may be helping to reduce anginal pain. While there is some evidence that bypass surgery may improve left ventricular functioning, according to the National Heart, Lung, and Blood Institute (1981), there are presently no statistically valid data to show that coronary artery surgery prolongs life.

New noninvasive diagnostic techniques such as echocardiography, cineangiography, radio nuclear scanning, computer-assisted tomography, and many others, are enabling doctors to diagnose CHD at an earlier stage. The medical profession may think their CHD patients are living longer; but in fact they may simply be getting diagnosed earlier.

Control of risk factors. This brings us to the possibility that it may be *preventive* measures that are responsible for the decline in CHD death rates. Due to an increased public awareness of the so-called risk factors, and genuine efforts among the medical profession to reduce these risk factors, it is possible that there has been a significant decline in the CHD death rate.

Different forms of cardiovascular disease are affected differently by the various risk factors. The most significant risk factor in peripheral vascular disease is cigarette smoking, while for cerebrovascular disease and strokes, high blood pressure creates the greatest risk. For coronary heart disease, there are three main risk factors: (1) blood cholesterol level—especially the level of low-density lipoprotein (LDL); (2) blood pressure; and (3) the number of cigarettes one smokes. These factors are more than additive; when more than one of them is present, the risks of CHD increase by a factor greater than the sum of the individual risks.

In the case of smoking, the life-threatening risk is reduced by ninety percent after quitting the habit for one year. Ten years after cessation of smoking, the increased risk of death from coronary heart disease is virtually totally eliminated. Thus heart attacks and death from this source are really quite simple to eliminate, by a simple act of willpower.

High blood pressure: a threat for strokes and heart disease. Thirty years ago people generally did not know they had high blood pressure until it was too late—that is, until they suffered a stroke or a heart attack. Nor was the treatment of hypertension very advanced. In the 1950s antihypertensive drugs came into use—the thiazide diuretics, methyldopa, and reserpine.

High blood pressure is very widespread among the American population. It has been estimated that one out of five American adults has hypertension. While hypertension is easy to detect, as recently as 1972 half the Americans with high blood pressure were unaware of the condition. In that year, with the initiation of the National High Blood Pressure Education Program, both medical professionals and the general public were made aware of the prevalence of hypertension, the ease of diagnosis, and the effectiveness of available treatment. Today only an estimated twenty percent of hypertensives are unaware of their condition. Whereas in 1972 only one eighth of all hypertensives—less than four million people—were receiving effective treatment, today over ten million Americans are being treated for high blood pressure.

As a result of this massive educational and treatment effort, the death rate from strokes has declined dramatically—by thirty-seven percent in the past ten years. This decline is undoubtedly largely due to the control of hypertension. While it is harder to establish a direct link between hypertension and heart attacks, the control of blood pressure is most likely also a factor in the prevention of coronary heart disease.

While a number of drugs are routinely used today to control blood pressure, we must remember that the simple dietary strategy of limiting sodium intake is an essential first step in the prevention of hypertension. We get all the sodium we need from our foods. There is no reason to add salt, either in cooking or at the table. By experimenting with herbs and spices, healthful garlic, and other flavors, you can introduce new zest into your meals while reducing the risk of heart attacks and stroke.

The cholesterol question: Does eating too much fat really clog our arteries? Ever since the cholesterol issue was first raised in the medical literature, there has been a great deal of confusion as to the degree to which dietary manipulation—namely, the reduction of saturated fats and cholesterol in the diet—can reduce the risk of heart attacks. More than sixty years ago it was shown that atherosclerosis could be produced in rabbits who were fed high-cholesterol diets, and coronary atherosclerosis was implicated as a causative factor in myocardial infarction, or heart attacks. More than thirty years ago, studies of various groups of people began to support the suspicion that dietary fat intake and atherosclerosis were somehow related.

While the medical profession has generally jumped on the bandwagon by encouraging Americans to reduce their consumption of cholesterol and saturated fats in an attempt to control blood cholesterol, and thereby hopefully atherosclerosis, the evidence to support this recommendation is still far from complete. An additional element that further confuses the picture is the eagerness of the food-processing industry to supply American consumers with dietary alternatives to the saturated fats that have allegedly been clogging up our arteries. We have been urged to consume more unsaturated oils in place of the saturated animal fats—certainly a reasonable suggestion on the face of it—and to use such food products as margarine in place of butter—a much more dubious recommendation!

Dangers of excessive polyunsaturates. It is probably true that most people will benefit from a substitution of unsaturated fats for saturated ones, and from a decrease in their total fat intake, if only because this will increase the amount of foods in the diet rich in the protective nutrients—namely, more fruits, vegetables, nuts, and whole grains. But it is dangerous to go overboard in the consumption of polyunsaturates. Polyunsaturated fats, like those found in most vegetable oils, have been shown to be subject to a process known as lipid peroxidation in the body, which is similar to the development of rancidity in oils. This process releases destructive free radicals or molecular fragments in the body which may be responsible for damage to our cells, manifested in such processes as increased wrinkling and perhaps even cancer.

Polyunsaturated vegetable oils, as they occur naturally in whole grains and seeds, are accompanied by protective antioxidants, most notably vitamin E. However, when vegetable oils are processed, they are usually robbed of their protective vitamin E content. The vitamin E removed from the seeds and grains is then packaged and sold to us separately, at a high price. Thus, the polyunsaturated oils we buy in the market, unless they have been *cold pressed*, are lacking in the protective vitamin E and other nutrients that might help to balance damaging lipid peroxidation and free radical formation.

When it comes to using margarine instead of butter, the case for polyunsaturates becomes even weaker. Margarine has been at least partially hydrogenated to give it solid form, thereby converting polyunsaturated fats into saturated ones of a particularly dangerous type. Margarine also contains additives and coloring agents which are highly suspect. Despite the exhortations of the food-processing industry, we really cannot recommend that you substitute this "junk food" for butter.

The confused cholesterol picture. In an article entitled "Unresolved Problems in the Diet-Heart Issue," Henry C. McGill, Jr., Alex McMahan, and Jamie Dollahite Wene (1981) summarize the current status of research on cholesterol and heart disease. It is clear that the issue remains unresolved. In some epidemiological studies, a correlation was found between dietary cholesterol and serum cholesterol concentrations. However, other studies have failed to show a relationship between saturated fat/cholesterol intake and myocardial infarction or death from coronary heart disease. Some studies have shown that our diet can be used to lower serum cholesterol, and yet even among people who were able to lower their serum cholesterol significantly through their diet, there is no conclusive evidence that there was a reduction in heart attacks and fatalities.

In studies with rhesus monkeys, there was evidence that not only could a high cholesterol diet be used to induce atherosclerotic lesions, but that with a reduction of the cholesterol in the diet, the animals' blood cholesterol could be lowered, and on autopsies these animals "had significantly less coronary atherosclerosis, less luminal stenosis, less fat in the coronary vessel wall, and less medial elastic lamina damage" (Levy 1981, p. 321; studies by Clarkson et al.). Such studies suggest that not only can blood cholesterol and atherogenesis be controlled through dietary means, but also that atherosclerotic lesions can actually be *reversed* when blood cholesterol levels are controlled through diet.

Such studies, of course, cannot be reproduced in humans. But the current popularity and stated success of such low-fat regimens as the Pritikin diet and associated exercise programs, indicates that dietary measures *may* help prevent fatal heart attacks.

Recent epidemiological evidence has suggested that high-density lipoprotein (HDL) is inversely related to atherosclerotic disease, while low-density lipoprotein, or LDL, is associated with atherosclerosis. According to recent research, each of these lipoprotein fractions can be influenced by dietary factors. We will see later in this chapter that alcohol consumption seems to *encourage* protective *HDL*. Other substances such as sugar, total carbohydrates, and starch, tend to *reduce* HDL levels.

Some investigators have suggested that it is not the levels of HDL or LDL in themselves that are important in determining the risk of cardiovascular disease, but that it is the LDL/HDL ratio. To make matters even more complicated, it now appears that HDL cholesterol, the desirable sort of lipoprotein, may *decrease* as the saturation of dietary fat decreases! This goes against the usual medical wisdom that saturated fat is bad for us.

Although high levels of HDL cholesterol and low LDL/HDL ratios are associated with less cardiovascular risk and less severe atherosclerosis, the relative importance of these two variables and whether manipulating them by diet actually changes a person's risk status are not known. However, we no longer can assume that plasma HDL cholesterol concentration is unresponsive to dietary lipid intake. In particular, some experiments indicate that it is influenced by dietary saturated fat.

(McGill et al. 1981, p. 169)

One final confusing issue in the cholesterol controversy is that in animals that are fed a high cholesterol/saturated fat diet, an adaptation phenomenon occurs, so that the serum cholesterol rises and then after about a year begins to decline. It is suspected that there may be similar adaptation responses to diet in humans. This may be why a modification of the diet does not reduce serum cholesterol to the degree that would be expected, and would account for some of the equivocal findings in human studies, since, as McGill et al. speculate, "subjects who had adapted would have only a limited capacity to reduce their serum cholesterol levels. . . . Adaptation to an atherogenic diet has been seen in animal experiments frequently enough to indicate that it is real, and to suggest that it is likely to occur also in humans" (McGill et al. 1981, p. 174).

A wise protective diet against atherosclerosis. We have certainly not yet arrived at the end of the long and tortuous road to the truth concerning dietary factors in the causation of coronary heart disease. For the time being, the wisest approach seems to be a middle-of-the-road one, reducing total fats and total proteins (specifically, meat proteins); increasing complex carbohydrates, particularly grain products and potatoes; decreasing refined sugars and starches, and substituting, moderately, unsaturated, or monosaturated oils for saturated fats. However, remember that polyunsaturated fat is contained in natural whole grains, and therefore using additional polyunsaturated fats beyond a very moderate amount, will result in an unbalanced fat intake.

Remember also, that high-fiber intake has been associated in epidemiological studies, with decreased incidence of coronary heart disease. By consuming more whole grains, fresh fruits, and vegetables, you also increase this important protective factor in your diet. In chapter 8 you will learn in detail how you can increase your fiber intake to protect against heart disease and many other health problems.

Have we been overlooking an important nutrient in the heart disease issue? In attempting to explain the decline in the CHD death rate, epidemiologists have generally singled out a shift in the American diet from saturated fat/cholesterol-bearing foods to unsaturated fats. We would like to suggest that the epidemiologists may have overlooked some other key nutrients.

You see, when people decrease their consumption of

foods high in saturated fats, they generally at the same time increase their consumption of other types of foods, such as whole grains, legumes, fresh fruits, and vegetables. It is possible that the decline in the CHD mortality rate is due *not* to a decrease in saturated fat/cholesterol intake, but rather to an *increase* in certain other dietary factors that are found in the newly substituted foods. We will now discuss one possible candidate for such a protective dietary factor—vitamin B_6.

A Banana a Day Keeps the Doctor Away: The B_6 Breakthrough

Bananas, avocados, lettuce, carrots, tomatoes, onions, kale, spinach, apples, sweet potatoes, and asparagus—what do these foods have in common? In descending order, all of these familiar foods are very rich in vitamin B_6 and low in the essential amino acid methionine, an essential amino acid, but only required in small quantities in our diet. These are most likely our most super-protective foods against the development of atherosclerosis, and later on, heart attacks.

The vitamin B_6-methionine theory, also known as the homocysteine theory, is the most exciting new area in the prevention of coronary heart disease. The potential of vitamin B_6 was known in medical research circles as long ago as 1948, when the pathologists James Rinehart and Louis Greenberg conducted a remarkable series of experiments at the University of California Medical School in San Francisco. They demonstrated conclusively, that monkeys who were fed diets deficient in vitamin B_6 rapidly developed atherosclerosis, while monkeys put on similar diets but deficient in the other B vitamins, did not develop atherosclerosis.

More recently the baton has been picked up by Kilmer McCully, M.D., Professor of Pathology at Harvard Medical School. Dr. McCully convincingly argues that a deficiency of vitamin B_6 in the diets of these animals, and likewise in humans, allows the amino acid methionine to become the very toxic chemical homocysteine. When vitamin B_6 is present, methionine's toxic breakdown product homocysteine, is converted into the nontoxic form called cystathionine.

Unlike cholesterol, which is normally present in our blood, homocysteine is not normally found in our blood. In plain English, homocysteine seems to cause atherosclerosis, and vitamin B_6 will prevent a buildup of this amino acid. Figure 1.2 shows schematically how this process takes place in the body.

Figure 1.2

How Vitamin B_6 Protects Against Homocysteine

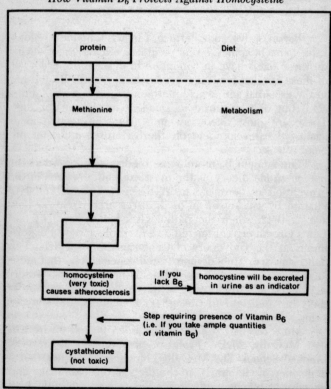

Source: Modified from Gruberg and Raymond 1979

Pieces of the homocysteine theory fell into place slowly. They were brilliantly described in a recent article entitled "Beyond Cholesterol: A New Theory of Arteriosclerosis" by Edward R. Gruberg and Stephen A. Raymond (1979):

> High levels of homocystine in human beings were first discovered by Dr. Nina Carson and her colleagues at the Royal Belfast Hospital for Sick Children in Northern Ireland. They were studying mental retardation, not atherosclerosis. Genetically inherited biochemical disorders are sometimes associated with retardation, and Carson and co-workers had been carrying out systematic biochemical screenings to determine families at risk.
>
> They had analyzed urine samples from two young sisters, Patricia and Pauline B. The girls, aged six and four respectively, were severely retarded. Patricia had a working vocabulary of twelve words and Pauline could not yet speak. Carson and colleagues reported in 1962 that these girls were excreting large amounts of homocystine in their urine. Homocystine is not normally found in the urine, and the two girls were the first known cases, although others were identified soon after Carson and her co-workers had reported the existence of the new disease, which they called homocystinuria. The link to atherosclerosis was established a few years later. Patricia B. died at age nine and a half. Autopsies on her and other young victims of homocystinuria (ages seven to thirteen) revealed extensive vascular disease and associated thromboses. It was as if the whole atherosclerotic process had occurred at a much accelerated pace, resulting in the early death of the patients.
>
> (Gruberg and Raymond 1979, pp. 61–62)

Dr. McCully reasons that the original injury in the coronary arteries is initiated by a deficiency of vitamin B_6. This concept seems to fit well with the heart disease statistics from around the world, because those nations where much fat and animal protein and few vegetables are eaten, seem to have the highest rates of coronary heart disease.

Referring to Table 1.3, you can see that the foods mentioned at the beginning of this section—mainly bananas, avocados, lettuce, carrots, and other vegetables—have a relatively high quantity of vitamin B_6 and are relatively low in the amino acid methionine. Foods such as beef are the reverse. They contain a great deal of methionine and only small quantities of vitamin B_6.

Table 1.3

B_6:Methionine Protective Ratios for Common Foods

Food	B_6:Methionine Ratio (x 1,000)	Food	B_6:Methionine Ratio (x 1,000)
Bananas	46	Lentils	3
Avocados	22	Peas	3
Oranges	22	Sunflower Seeds	3
Lettuce	17	Toasted Wheat Germ	3
Carrots	15	Beef Liver	2
Onions	10	Chickpeas	2
Potatoes	10	Corn	2
Kale	9	Peanuts	2
Apples	7.5	Soybeans	2
Spinach	7	Walnuts	2
Sweet Potatoes	7	Chicken	1
Asparagus	5	Salmon	1
Cauliflower	5	Beef	.9
Turnip Greens	5	Mushrooms	.7
Broccoli	4	Cod	.5
Brewer's Yeast	3	Eggs	.3

Remember, vitamin B_6 or pyridoxine, is a water-soluble vitamin. It is carried mainly in foods that are rich in water; and the more fat in the diet, the less of this vitamin we get. So if we eat diets rich in meats and fats, which are already deficient in B_6, and if in addition we rely on processed foods in which the vitamin B_6 is almost totally destroyed, we will not be getting enough pyridoxine to protect ourselves against the large amounts of methionine that we get from the animal products. If this is true, then you can see why a change in the American diet—reducing the intake of total fats and substituting unsaturated for saturated fats (that is, substituting more vegetable products for meats and animal fats), might have resulted in a decline in the coronary disease death rate—*although the explanation generally offered, namely that cholesterol had been reduced in the diet, might not have told the whole story*.

Can we reverse the original lesion? As has been suggested in animal studies of cholesterol-controlled diets, Dr. McCully believes that we can reverse atherosclerotic lesions—but he believes this is done through a sufficient intake of vitamin B_6. He is quoted in *Prevention* magazine as follows:

> Moses M. Suzman of Johannesburg, South Africa carried out a study on 17 patients with coronary artery disease. Animal protein was reduced to approximately one-quarter to one-half of their customary intake and each patient received 100 mg. pyridoxine daily with a potent preparation of vitamin B complex. The patients were observed for an average of 13 months. All patients claimed a notable increase in exercise tolerance with complete or partial relief of angina, a gain in energy and a heightened sense of well-being. Glucose tolerance increased to almost normal in two of the patients who were diabetic. This study suggests that the lesions may be partially reversible with B_6.
>
> (Kinderlehrer 1979, p. 144)

B_6 also influences platelets. As is so often the case with valuable protective nutrients, it appears that vitamin B_6 may help in yet another way to prevent heart attacks. According to research by Kornecki and Feinberg (1980), pyridoxal phosphate, one of the active forms of vitamin B_6, inhibits platelet aggregation, or clumping, which is an underlying process in atherosclerosis. Platelets, the cells which control blood clotting, normally flow freely through the bloodstream. When they reach a place where the blood vessel is damaged, they attach to the spot and release adenosine diphosphate (ADP), a platelet-aggregating chemical. The platelets in the blood then begin to adhere to one another and form a clot that can block the flow through the damaged vessel, which can result in heart attacks. The prestigious British medical journal, *Lancet*, suggests a protective dosage of B_6 against platelet aggrega-

tion: "Moderate doses of vitamin B_6 (say, 40 mg. a day) may suffice to alter the natural history of such a process" (Mazer 1982, p. 22).

A safe and inexpensive supplement. Remember this: An excess intake of vitamin B_6 is excreted very rapidly, and this vitamin is extremely safe. The toxic dose of pyridoxine is approximately ten grams per day, which makes it about as toxic as common table salt. Again we see that eating simple foods and supplementing with relatively inexpensive B vitamins, may spell the difference between life and death.

Additional Pieces of the Heart Disease Puzzle

There are other factors in the development—or lack of development—of coronary heart disease that are often overlooked in the mad study of cholesterol and fat. Among these other factors are alcohol, garlic, and angiotoxins.

Good news for moderate drinkers. The question of the relative benefits of drinking wine and other alcoholic beverages has been debated since the first grape was fermented. The opinion that alcohol could be a major factor in the development of atherosclerosis and coronary heart disease became most pronounced during the nineteenth century. The tide turned when one shrewd observer by the name of Cabot, showed his skeptical physician friends that the incidence of atherosclerotic lesions in autopsies on patients with a history of alcoholism, was usually very low. It seems that in medicine there are always at least two differing opinions, and so a crafty worker named Wilens suggested that the low incidence of atherosclerosis in chronic alcoholism, was probably due to the fact that the alcoholics in the autopsy room were usually dead at a younger age (Baraona and Lieber 1979). Still another group of investigators claimed that the rarity of myocardial infarction in people with cirrhosis was a statistical fallacy based on the likelihood that two fatal diseases would not be found together.

In the midst of all this, a very wise worker by the name of M. A. Ruffer, showed that atheroma (the fatty degeneration or thickening of large arterial walls) occurred frequently in devout Muslims whose religion prohibited the use of alcoholic beverages. This finding was reported back in 1911 in the *Journal of Pathology and Bacteriology*, in an article entitled "On Arterial Lesions Found in Egyptian Mummies."

More recently, the epidemiologists have entered the controversy over alcohol and heart disease. A definite negative correlation between alcohol consumption and CHD was shown in several, but not all, of their studies—which tends to revive the hope that alcohol has a protective effect against atherosclerosis and ischemic heart disease.

Unfortunately we do not have any reliable human studies, but several classic animal studies indicate that alcohol is an effective way to reduce our risk of developing heart disease. Eberhard fed a high-cholesterol diet to rabbits for approximately twenty weeks. He found that adding twenty-five percent ethanol to the animals' drinking water produced a significant increase in the concentrations of cholesterol in both the liver and the plasma; but atherosclerotic lesions of the aorta and the cholesterol content of the vessel wall were both reduced (Baraona and Lieber 1979). We repeat: By adding twenty-five percent ethanol to the drinking water, cholesterol was increased in the liver and in the plasma, but *decreased* in the walls of the vessel, and lesions of the aorta were decreased.

The most recent and reliable studies have been done in rhesus monkeys. By the way, atherosclerosis has been produced in these unfortunate animals by a typical "table-prepared" American diet. One of the best studies of the effect of alcohol in these animals was performed by Rudel and co-workers (1979). They took nineteen monkeys and divided them up into several groups. The diets contained low-versus high-cholesterol levels, and no ethanol or ethanol as thirty-six percent of the calories which were substituted for an equivalent amount of carbohydrate in the diet. After feeding these diets for approximately a year and a half, blood samples were drawn from the monkeys for lipoprotein analysis upon autopsies. The authors concluded that ethanol very definitely and significantly decreased the atherosclerosis found in the aorta and coronary arteries compared with the nonethanol-fed groups. If you were to look at the photomicrographs taken of the coronary arteries of the two groups of animals, you would probably run out for a glass of wine. On the left side of the page you would see the coronary artery of an animal fed a high-cholesterol diet alone, and you would notice that the artery had in fact a rather thick plaque surrounding most of the circumference of the vessel. On the right side you would see a cross section of the coronary artery of the monkey fed the high-cholesterol diet *plus ethanol,* and true enough, the artery has only a small lesion in one area.

HDLs and LDLs. Now remember, there are two types of lipoproteins—*HDLs,* or high-density lipoproteins—which are the *protective* ones; and *LDLs,* or low-density lipoproteins, which are associated with an increased risk of heart disease. We want to *raise* our HDLs and *decrease* our LDLs. Rudel and co-workers conclude that "the alcohol-induced modification resulted in an LDL of lower molecular weight and in higher HDL levels. Ethanol appeared to prevent much of the cholesterol-induced coronary artery atherosclerosis and ethanol-fed animals had less aortic atherosclerosis than those not receiving ethanol."

While the authors caution us that cause-and-effect relationships should not be drawn from this experiment, they state that "the results strongly suggest the possibility that dietary ethanol and cholesterol are influencing the extent of atherosclerosis through their effect on plasma LDL composition and on HDL levels." They also point out that while adding alcohol to our diets might have a beneficial effect in reducing our chance of developing coronary atherosclerosis, it might *not* protect our *cerebral* circulation! Also, they were unable to determine the full effect of alcohol on the liver and other organs. But the direction they are heading in is a hopeful one. What they are seeking is the *lowest level* of ethanol that would reduce our risk of coronary heart disease, but without destroying our brains and liver. In their study, 36 percent of the calories had to be ethanol in order to have a protective effect—that is, over one third of the diet was in the form of ethanol!

In a different study, Phillips and her colleagues (1981)

found that protective HDL cholesterol was *increased* in both sexes as the quantity of dietary ethanol increased, while the amount of HDL cholesterol *decreased* as the number of cigarettes smoked daily increased and as the body fat ratio increased. This large-scale epidemiological study was conducted on a defined population sample of 9,000 Caucasian men and 1,400 Caucasian women between the ages of 20 and 64 who were employees of the Southern Pacific Railroad working in the San Francisco Bay and Sacramento-Roseville areas of California.

These recent studies tend to confirm the work done during the past decade on the same subject. Back in 1974, Klatsky and co-workers (1974) stated that in the 464 patients studied, there was a statistically significant negative association between the amount of alcohol that one consumed and a subsequent first heart attack. This study was well controlled for cigarette smoking and five other risk factors. Interestingly, those people who had a heart attack generally came from two groups—those who were teetotalers and those who were heavy drinkers. Those who were light or moderate drinkers did better.

Most scientists are supercautious, and these researchers are no exception.

> It thus seems fair to say that there is some clinical and experimental evidence for a beneficial effect of alcohol on the coronary circulation. But the case for this is far from convincing. Since there is a considerable amount of evidence for a harmful effect of alcohol on myocardial cells and since it is not possible to predict which individuals are susceptible to alcoholic heart disease, damage to the heart has to be considered as one of the many serious hazards of consuming large amounts of alcohol. The use of small amounts of alcohol might not be harmful to myocardial cells. Although the findings of a statistically significant negative association between use of alcohol and a first myocardial infarction cannot at this time be interpreted as proof of a protective effect of alcohol on the coronary vessels, this happy possibility does exist.
>
> (Klatsky, Friedman, and Siegelaub 1974, p. 300)

Other human studies have more definitely shown that ethanol does in fact *decrease* the risk of atherosclerosis. Stason and co-workers (1976) reported that those people who drank six or more drinks per day (!) had a lower risk of developing a heart attack:

> The data of this study indicate that the rate of nonfatal myocardial infarction in regular, heavy users of alcoholic beverages is no higher than in nonusers; if anything, it seems to be lower. . . .
> The current study provides evidence against a positive association between alcohol consumption and the risk of myocardial infarction, and tends to corroborate previous evidence of a negative association.

Of interest to the athletically inclined is a recent report in *Nutrition Reviews*, "Alcohol Consumption and High-Density Lipoprotein Cholesterol in Marathon Runners" (1981) that claims that "a positive association which cannot be explained by the effect of vigorous exercise appears to exist between alcohol consumption and high-density lipoprotein cholesterol levels." The subjects consisted of 90 male physicians, aged 27 to 68, who participated in the 1979 Doctors' Marathon in Boston. This study showed that mean HDL levels were about 51.7 mg./dl. in the 14 physicians who drank no alcohol, 53.9 mg./dl. in the 52 who consumed up to six ounces of alcohol weekly, and 61.5 mg./dl. in the 24 doctors who drank six to eighteen ounces of alcohol every week. While the author of the article states that these results "do not provide a basis for recommending that nondrinkers adopt the habit of moderate alcohol consumption, it might be useful to examine HDL-cholesterol in sedentary moderate drinkers to evaluate a possible synergistic effect of exercise and alcohol."

Interestingly, the amount of wine consumed in the United States has significantly increased in the past two decades, just as the heart disease rate has declined. We are informed by the Economic Research Department of the Wine Institute of San Francisco, that the per capita consumption of wine has shown a steady climb:

1960	0.91 gallons per person
1970	1.31 gallons per person
1980	2.12 gallons per person

Finally, for those of you who wonder what "moderate" means with regard to alcohol, the venerable British medical establishment has defined that one for us—it is equal to approximately seven ounces of alcohol per day or two pints of beer or one liter of wine!

A note about alcoholism. In our opinion, alcoholism is symptomatic of a complex of nutritional deficiencies. Dr. Roger Williams, a highly respected nutritionist, has devoted an entire book to this problem (Williams 1981). He suggests a regimen of a multivitamin/mineral preparation and increased quantities of the amino acid glutamine. We also recommend strongly that a "preventive pill" (that is, a high-potency vitamin/mineral formula) be taken. By eating the foods suggested in each chapter and avoiding the highly refined carbohydrates which tend to *increase* the demand for stimulants and alcohol, the problem drinker will slowly experience a diminished craving. Remember that alcohol, in moderation, can be a great salve of old age.

Garlic. Dr. Arun Bordia has been producing some interesting work in India over the last few years. In a study published in the *American Journal of Clinical Nutrition* (1981), Dr. Bordia has definitively shown that garlic has a cholesterol-lowering effect. Two groups of individuals are described. In the first group 20 healthy volunteers were fed garlic for six months and then followed for another two months without garlic; it was found that this foodstuff significantly *lowered* serum cholesterol and triglycerides while *raising* protective HDLs. The second group, consisting of 62 patients who had a previous history of coronary heart disease and elevated serum cholesterol, was divided into two subgroups. Subgroup 1 was fed garlic for ten months, while subgroup 2 served as a control, being fed no garlic. Again garlic was found to *decrease* the serum cholesterol, triglycerides, and LDLs, while *increasing* the HDLs. The author concluded that the essential oil of garlic had shown a distinct hypolipidemic (blood-fat-lowering) action both in healthy individuals and in patients with a previous history of heart disease.

How much garlic does it take? In this study, the garlic was given in the form of its essential oil. A 150-pound man was given about 15 milligrams of garlic oil, which corresponds to about 30 grams of raw garlic clove (about 1.2 ounces per day). During the six months of the garlic feeding the serum cholesterol decreased by about 17 percent, and serum triglycerides decreased by about 20 percent. Both of these changes are seen as statistically significant.

This study tends to confirm what people of the Mediterranean have intuitively known and practiced since antiquity; namely, that garlic (and as we saw earlier, a little wine) can go a long way toward reducing our risk of developing heart disease.

Recalling the extremely protective nature of vitamin B_6-rich foods, particularly those high in B_6 and low in the amino acid methionine, we saw that onions were among the most protective foods, with a ratio of 10 (meaning that the food has 10,000 times more B_6 than methionine). Since garlic is the same botanical genus as onions, namely *Allium*, we can expect that including such foods as garlic and onions (and, as we saw earlier, carrots, bananas, kale, spinach, sweet potatoes, asparagus, cauliflower, turnip greens, broccoli, and so on) in your diet, will serve to reduce your risk of developing atherosclerosis and coronary heart disease.

Angiotoxins. So far we have emphasized *deficiencies* of certain nutrients in the causation of coronary heart disease. This concept is a reversal of earlier trends in modern pathology, which had prepared us to believe that the immediate cause of any disease must be the result of some positive factor, such as a parasite or a toxin—a poison, the so-called *materia morbi*. While the development of heart disease seems to be ameliorated by the inclusion of these protective nutrients, in fact, there may be something to the idea that cholesterol-laden foods, when they are spontaneously broken down into their toxic derivatives, develop into highly atherogenic substances.

We have already outlined the cholesterol controversy

in some detail. Some recent studies indicate that *pure* cholesterol is not atherogenic; but *oxidized* cholesterol and spontaneously produced *toxic derivatives* of cholesterol may be highly atherogenic. What happens is that when cholesterol-containing foods are left out in the air, oxidation products are generated, and these could be some of the most important dietary factors in the development of atherosclerosis, and later, of coronary heart disease.

Taylor and co-workers (1979), in a recent paper titled "Spontaneously Occurring Angiotoxic Derivatives of Cholesterol," point out that almost all of the studies done on the effects of cholesterol are faulty because in the majority of cases the cholesterol used in these experimental diets most likely contained "significant quantities of oxidized sterols that have a striking lethal effect on aortic smooth muscle cells." These researchers strongly suggest that pure cholesterol is not atherogenic, and that only when cholesterol is broken down through oxidation to produce toxic derivatives—that is, when cholesterol-containing foods are stored at room temperature—that only then may they become highly atherogenic.

These workers recommend that until some changes are made in the means by which cholesterol-containing foods are stored, certain common food items should be avoided. Of particular concern are commercially available powdered dehydrated foods, such as powdered egg yolks, powdered eggs, powdered milk, and retail foods that contain dried whey, which is made from whole milk. Even powdered custard mix or pancake mixes, which do not often list the fact that they contain powdered whole milk or powdered eggs in their ingredients, should be avoided. According to the present methods of dehydrating foods, many angiotoxic derivatives are formed owing to oxidation and the chemical alteration of cholesterol.

Future techniques for safely preserving such foods might include storing them in a very cold place under nitrogen gas or in a vacuum environment, or adding appropriate antioxidants.

Other foods which have often had their cholesterol broken down into toxic derivatives include smoked fish, smoked meat, smoked sausages, and even some cheeses, particularly those that are exposed to the elements for long periods of time during processing and then stored only at room temperature.

Eggs, angiotoxins, and heart attacks. So much has been written about the humble egg, which we consider to be one of the most important superfoods—and by the way, a food which should *not* be excluded from the diet—that we feel that quoting directly from Dr. Taylor's article is in order:

The egg, which has 250 to 300 mg of cholesterol in each yolk, should be mentioned. Its defamation as a large source of cholesterol began with Anitschkow's studies (Germany, 1912–1913). The description of Anitschkow's experiments provides reasonable assurance that the sterols in the eggs he fed had ample opportunity to become oxidized.

The fertilized egg when freshly laid contains all essential ingredients for normal maturation of the chick. The intact egg can be stored in a 36°F refrigerator for several weeks and remain viable and subsequently hatched. Today the egg industry refrigerates their eggs (unfertilized) shortly after they are laid and delivers the eggs to retail stores within a week, where they are also refrigerated. *Thus today's egg industry puts eggs in consumers' hands that are probably free of spontaneous degradation products* [our italics]. This was probably not the case before 1940, before farm electrification made it possible to have continuous egg production throughout the year; illumination of henneries for 14 to 16 hours per day during the winter months, when days are short, stimulates hens to lay eggs as if they were long summer days, in midwinter. Cyclical egg production (essentially no egg production during winter months) and earlier storage procedures, before the 1940s, could conceivably have permitted degradation of cholesterol in egg yolks after normally present antioxidants such as glutathione, vitamin C, and vitamin E were depleted in eggs stored at near room temperature for four to six months.

There still remains, of course, the proper preparation of even fresh eggs. Heat, in the presence of oxygen, can induce oxidation. Whether this potential is real needs to be ascertained. Interestingly, Pollak in

1958 demonstrated that the response of serum cholesterol levels varied when differently prepared egg diets were fed to rabbits. *Fried or hard boiled* eggs produced the *highest* serum cholesterol levels (ten to fourteen times greater than the pre-experimental level), *scrambled or baked* eggs caused elevation of serum cholesterol to six to seven times the pre-experimental level, *raw or soft boiled* eggs only increased serum cholesterol levels three to four times the pre-experimental level [our italics]. The results suggest that the nature or the content of cholesterol in eggs might be changed by different methods of preparation.

Thus the egg, when poached or soft-boiled, is relatively safe from the cholesterol standpoint, and extremely beneficial in terms of the other important protective nutrients it provides. Any foods containing cholesterol should be stored in a very well-sealed container and refrigerated or kept frozen. This means that you should not leave your butter, cheese, Parmesan cheese, meats, or any other dairy products around at room temperature if you want to avoid creating dangerous oxidation products which could induce atherogenesis and speed up the development of heart disease.

Rate Your Protective Factors Against Heart Disease

We now have some strong coordinates in the heart disease puzzle.* By using the following "building block" and ranking yourself for these *positive protective factors* (instead of the negative risk factors so widely used), you can calculate your own progress in increasing your heart protective profile.

---

*I considered an entire chapter on a method used to *reverse* atherosclerosis called Chelation. However, the conclusions are not *yet* sufficient for me to recommend this therapy, although it appears to be very promising. Further, this technique, while a far more sensible alternative to coronary bypass surgery, is *not* a nutritional therapy and therefore not in the scope of this book.

Building Block #1:

"Don't Lose Heart!"
Your Protective Factors Against Heart Disease

Eats B$_6$-rich foods (See p. 15 & p. 18) 10 points	Eats high-fiber foods (15–25 grams) (See p. 14 & chapter 8) 9 points	Does not smoke (See p. 9) 8 points
Fats no more than 30% of diet (See p. 10) 7 points	Exercises vigorously at least three times weekly (See p. 60) 6 points	Does not add salt to foods (See p. 10) 5 points
Takes vitamin B$_6$ supplement (25–100 mg.) (See p. 20) 4 points	Avoids angiotoxins (See p. 26) 3 points	Drinks wine (See p. 20) 2 points

Total the points for your present protective factors.

Your Score
Block #1 _____

To page 46

for your next building block

2

ELUDING THE BIG C:

Diet and Cancer Prevention

For years it has been implied in the health food literature that certain foods can induce cancer when eaten to excess—for example, foods containing nitrites, which convert to potent carcinogens in the body, or high-fat diets, which are implicated in the development of breast cancer. On the other hand, these sources say, certain foods such as vegetables and fruits rich in vitamins A and C and bioflavonoids, as well as grains rich in fiber, can protect us against cancer. The official medical platform has been that diet has little effect on the development or outcome of cancer. Now, though, some of the most respected and staid medical researchers are beginning to see the light.

The long-term study recently published by the National Academy of Sciences, is a case in point. Here, a highly conservative group of scientists studying the etiology of cancer from a multidisciplinary approach, concluded that high-fat diets are associated with an increased incidence of this dread disease.

Another recent study of major proportions was conducted by Dr. Richard Doll, who is the honorary director of the Imperial Cancer Research Fund Cancer Epidemiology and Clinical Trials Unit at Oxford, England, and his coauthor Richard Peto, a cancer researcher at Oxford University (1981). Their study categorically states that of all elements contributing to cancer, *"the largest risk is due to dietary factors"* [our italics]. Even more significantly, the study states that "there is quite good evidence that cancer is *largely an avoidable* (although not necessarily a modern) *disease"* [our italics]. Our purpose in this chapter is to show you which dietary factors are particularly important in promoting and in retarding the development of cancer, and which environmental factors are also important in avoiding this dread disease.

Diet—the Leading Factor in Cancer Deaths

Looking at Table 2.1, you can see that of all the factors related to cancer mortality, diet is at the top of the

Table 2.1

*Proportions of Cancer Deaths
Attributed to Various Factors*

Factor or class of factors	Percent of all cancer deaths (best estimate)
Diet	35
Tobacco	30
Infection	10?
Reproductive and sexual behavior	7
Occupation	4
Alcohol	3
Geophysical factors	3
Pollution	2
Medicines and medical procedures	1
Food additives	<1
Industrial products	<1
Unknown	?

Source: Doll and Peto 1981, p. 1256

list, and accounts for thirty-five percent. This is followed
by the use of tobacco, then (questionably) by infection,
next by reproductive and sexual behavior, occupational
hazards, alcohol, and after these, by additional factors
such as geophysical factors, pollution, medicines and medical procedures, industrial products, and unknown causes.

Cancer results from nutritional deficiency. This thirty-
five percent rate of cancer causation due to dietary factors
is presently quite speculative and is not really firmly nailed
down. But it's important to remember that diet has its
most important effect not as a result of your *taking in*
potential carcinogens—although these must certainly be
guarded against—but rather as a result of the *lack of
protective factors* in your diet such as vitamins A and C,
the trace element selenium, and other micronutrients which
act to inhibit the development of cancer. Just as we observed in the case of heart disease, the changes that have
occurred in the Western diet may be responsible for the
present "cancer epidemic." But cancer may prove to be a
disease of *malnutrition* rather than the result of some
disease-producing substance or substances in our food.

Hidden Cancers in Food

The relationship between diet and cancer is complex
and many-sided. Let's first look at those dietary elements
known or suspected to incite cancer, and then see which
protective dietary factors are often *missing* from our foods.

Naturally occurring carcinogens in foods. Some foods
actually contain cancer-causing substances. This category
includes foods such as the bracken fern, which is eaten in
Japan. Interestingly and unfortunately, the Japanese who
eat bracken fern on a daily basis have three times as great
a risk of developing cancer of the esophagus as do the
Japanese who avoid it. Other naturally occurring carcinogens include cycasin, which is found in the cycad nut, and
methylhydrazine, found in the wild mushroom *Gyromitra
esculenta*—dietary items not commonly found in the average diet.

While these cancer-causing foods are not commonly

eaten, they are mentioned to show that carcinogens do exist in nature. More to the point of prevention are those carcinogens *produced* in very common dietary items; these must be avoided like the plague. Let's look at some of the ways that these substances can be produced in our food.

Cooking methods make a difference. Carcinogens produced during cooking must definitely not be overlooked. It has been known for years, for example, that benzopyrene and other polycyclic hydrocarbons are often produced by pyrolysis when fish or meat is smoked or broiled, or when any food is fried in fat that is repeatedly used (such as deep-fried chicken, fish, or french fries). Charcoal broiling steaks also produces powerful mutagens, and we seriously recommend that the backyard barbecue pit be filled with soil and turned into a planter.

Aflatoxin and other contaminants in stored foods. Another category of cancer-causing agents often comes to us from stored foods. Aflatoxin is a product of the fungus *Aspergillus flavus*. This fungus often contaminates peanuts and other carbohydrate foods which are stored in hot and humid climates, and it is believed that it contributes to the development of liver cancer in many tropical countries. In fact, aflatoxins are among the most powerful known agents causing liver cancer in some animal species. They are most likely equally dangerous for human beings because our liver cells contain the enzymes needed to produce the metabolic products that appear responsible for *Aspergillus's* cancer-causing activity.

In certain parts of Africa where primary liver cancer is very widespread, a direct relationship has been made with people who eat the greatest amount of dietary aflatoxin from peanuts and other stored foods. This disease tends to affect people who have been infected with hepatitis B virus, and so it seems likely that where aflatoxin is present in large quantities in the diet, both it and the hepatitis B virus work together somehow and multiply each other's carcinogenic effects.

While liver cancer is a fairly rare disease in the United States, and accounts for less than one percent of all cancer deaths in people under the age of sixty-five, it would still be wise to pay careful attention to the nuts and nut products that you buy, rejecting any which seem to be slightly rancid. Of course, with peanut butter the only assurance is to buy a high-quality brand and hope that the butter is not made from old, aflatoxin-infected peanuts. Another dietary route of concern would be dairy products that might be affected with aflatoxin if the cattle ate contaminated feed.

Other fungi in stored foods, such as *Penicillium*, *Fusarium*, and other *Aspergillus* species, have also been targeted by some scientists as naturally occurring chemical carcinogens to watch out for.

Nitrites and nitrosamines. Another way that diet can influence the development of cancer is by assisting in the formation of carcinogens inside the body, particularly N-nitroso compounds. These substances are the most powerful chemical carcinogens ever tested in the laboratory, and the development of even small amounts in the human body as a result of dietary intake, can be a serious danger. These compounds are found in very minute quantities in our gastric juice, and may be produced in the digestive tract or possibly in an infected bladder as a result of a reaction between nitrites and various nitrosable compounds such as secondary amines. This bit of chemistry would be assisted by formaldehyde, which is sometimes used to preserve foods, or by thiocyanate ions which could occur in our bodies from tobacco smoke.

But here's the good news. In order for this reaction to occur, a mildly acid medium is required, or the presence of certain bacteria. It is inhibited by antioxidants. The safest thing to do is to make sure that you have an adequate intake of antioxidants such as vitamin C with all of your meals—either from foods themselves or from vitamin supplements.

Nitrites and nitrosable compounds occur naturally in many foods, particularly in meat and fish. They are also frequently ingested through the drugs that we may take or in pesticide residues, and they may even be formed in our large intestine from amino acids. Nitrites are very often added to foods such as frankfurters, sausages, ham, bologna, and salami as preservatives, flavor enhancers, and coloring agents. But even if we were to avoid added nitrites in our foods—which we should do at all costs to reduce this risk—the most significant source of nitrite actually comes from within our bodies from the production of nitrates. Nitrates may occur naturally in vegetables and sometimes in drinking water, and are added to some foods as a preservative.

But there is a silver lining. We certainly don't want to avoid vegetables, which although they are the main source of nitrates in most of our diets, nevertheless protect against the development of stomach and other cancers, to a greater extent than they cause the development of these diseases. This is probably because the plants contain vitamins A, C, and others, as well as dietary fiber, which serve to "overpower" the negative effects of nitrates.

By-products of high-fat, high-meat diets. Our diet can also affect us via the production and excretion of cholesterol and bile acids. Certain fats that we eat can contribute to the development of carcinogens in our bodies because they increase the amount of cholesterol metabolites and bile acids in our feces. Larger amounts of these suspect substances are found in the feces of patients with cancer or adenomatous polyps in the colon than in the feces of patients with other diseases or in healthy control subjects. Also, the amounts of these dangerous substances in the feces can be experimentally increased in humans by high-fat, high-meat diets. By studying populations around the world, it has been found that two of these harmful substances, deoxycholic and lithocholic acids, are often found in the feces of populations on a Western type of high-fat, high-meat diet, in whom colorectal cancer is common, whereas in the feces of populations on characteristic Asian or African diets, these substances are rare. It is also known that dietary cholesterol or bile acids given with small doses of carcinogens, seem to speed up the development of tumors of the large intestine in experimental animals.

Protective Nutrients

How antioxidants protect against cancer. Rulon W. Rawson (1980), director of the Bonneville Center for Research on Cancer Cause and Prevention of the University of Utah, tells us that a daily dose of four grams of vitamin C decreased by almost fifty percent, the mutagens found in the feces of high-meat, high-fat eaters! This is another good reason to supplement your diet. Even more impressive is his report that "vitamin C plus vitamin E causes the complete absence of mutagens in the stool" (Rawson 1980, p. 19).

The reason these vitamins protect us is because many carcinogens must first be oxidized to yield "metabolically activated" intermediates before they can damage the cells of the body. In addition to simply adding ordinary oxygen in the normal cell processes, there are other mechanisms whereby oxidation and peroxidation occur, such as via oxidative free radicals or through so-called excited molecular oxygen. The scientists reason that certain carcinogens might be "defused" if various parts of our bodies were permeated with antioxidants, free radical traps, or substances which quench molecular excitation. One of the best ways for trapping free radicals and peroxidases consists of vitamin E and a selenium-containing enzyme working together. It is well-known that selenium and vitamin E definitely protect laboratory animals against carcinogens under rigorous experimental conditions.

We must point out however, that high levels of selenium can be toxic in and of themselves, and so the solution is not to take megadoses of selenium, but rather to get your selenium from natural sources—from such selenium-rich foods as asparagus, garlic, and whole wheat products, as well as mushrooms. If a supplement is taken, be certain that it contains no more than fifty micrograms of selenium in addition to your dietary sources. We repeat again; this is an extremely toxic trace metal and megadoses are to be avoided. If you or someone you know is suddenly losing their hair and also happens to be consuming selenium-potent vitamin supplements, discontinue the selenium and see if the hair loss stops. Other symptoms of selenium poisoning in humans include certain types of dermatitis, fatigue, dizziness, and loss of the fingernails; the latter was noted as long ago as in the time of Marco Polo, who in his journeys observed that his horses' hooves fell off when the animals grazed on plants from certain soils—soils which we now understand to have been overly rich in selenium.*

Vitamin E is another wonderful antioxidant and very easy to supplement with, although it is the most expensive of the vitamins. Finally, carrots and certain dark green leafy vegetables which contain beta-carotene, are of nutritional importance because they effectively quench the energy of excited oxygen which can eventually damage the cells of the body. Remember, one molecule of beta-carotene is converted in the human intestine into two molecules of vitamin A, and while it is not known precisely whether beta-carotene by itself quenches the oxygen as a protective mechanism, it also may work simply because it is a precursor of vitamin A, which is known to have a protective effect.

Among other sources of free radicals in the body we must warn against the excessive consumption of polyunsaturated fats. Many people, in an attempt to avoid high blood cholesterol and atherosclerosis, have switched from a diet high in saturated animal fats to one relatively high in polyunsaturated vegetable oils. In a process known as lipid peroxidation, unsaturated fats react with oxygen in the body's cells and release free radicals. While antioxidant vitamins E and C and the mineral selenium will help protect against free radical damage (vitamin E occurs naturally in seeds and grains that are rich in polyunsaturated oils, but *not* in the refined oils you buy in the market), we must still recommend that your consumption of *all* fats be kept low, and that you restrict your intake of polyunsaturates. An authority on aging, Dr. Denham Harman of the University of Nebraska College of Medicine, has warned that the concentrated use of polyunsaturates can have a definite, marked life-shortening effect. Free radical damage, from polyunsaturates and other sources including radiation, cigarette smoke, and other environmental sources, can produce premature skin wrinkling, cell damage, and genetic damage, as well as promote the development of cancer.

*One of the strongest and most concise scientific papers on the benefits of selenium and other free radical scavengers in preventint carcinogenesis is by F. C. Johnson (1982); see bibliography.

Vitamin A deficiency and cancer. Each month new evidence accumulates in the scientific literature that vitamin A might be one of our most potent tools in the prevention of cancer. When we say vitamin A we mean retinol as well as the related retinoids and various esters of vitamin A. All these substances seem to reduce the conversion of altered cells into a pathologic tumor. In addition to animal studies, some limited human studies using stored blood samples (Kark et al. 1981; Wald et al. 1980) suggest that vitamin A protects against the development of cancer. However, it's important to remember that through some unknown means our body itself controls the level of vitamin A in the blood, without depending on supplementation. Remember, we are talking about *circulating* levels of vitamin A, not stored vitamin A precursors in the liver. In other words, we can take megadoses of vitamin A and still see very little increase of vitamin A levels in the blood. As Doll and Peto conclude, "The simple expedient of adding much more vitamin A than normal to the diet has little effect on the level of vitamin A in the blood, and so the observation that blood vitamin A levels are inversely correlated with cancer does not automatically suggest that dietary supplementation with vitamin A will materially affect cancer risks in developed countries" (Doll and Peto 1981, p. 1232). Of course, in underdeveloped countries where vitamin A intake is marginal to begin with, chronic vitamin A deficiency may increase the risk of cancer. The consumption of vitamin-A-rich foods or the use of supplementary vitamin A could be an extremely important preventive measure. To aid you in your diet planning, Table A.1 in the Appendix lists some foods rich in vitamin A.

Fiber is a powerful protective factor. Most of us now appreciate the importance of dietary fiber, both in promoting bowel regularity and in reducing the amount of cholesterol and bile acids. So important is dietary fiber that we will be discussing its many benefits in a separate chapter.

Denis Burkitt may be considered the great popularizer of dietary fiber usage in the Western world. In his ground-breaking papers in the late 1960s and early 1970s, Burkitt shared his observations that a number of intestinal diseases that seem to be common in Western nations are rare in rural India and Africa, where natural unmilled grains are consumed to a greater extent, and where also feces tend to be more frequent, are bulkier, and softer. His hypothesis was of course roundly unsupported in the beginning, and international statistics correlating cancer deaths against food supplies were shown to be incompatible with his theory.

At that time, however, the detractors of the fiber theory were looking only at foods containing *crude* fiber. Since then, work has been done which characterized "dietary fiber" in a much broader sense. Dietary fiber in general, which is defined as "remnants of the plant cell wall not hydrolyzed by human alimentary enzymes," occurs in whole wheat in five times greater quantity than simple crude fiber. Dietary fiber includes cellulose, lignins, hexose, pentose, and uronic acid polymers. Each of these components of dietary fiber has different effects inside the body.

Of particular interest are the pentose polymers, which are very abundant in unrefined grains and occur to a lesser extent in other vegetables. Case-control studies have shown that patients with cancer of the large bowel have generally consumed such cereals and vegetables less frequently than the average. The pentose polymers tend to produce soft, bulky stools—not solely because they have a water-binding capacity, but also because they increase the amount of certain intestinal bacteria. (An astonishingly large proportion of the stool bulk is made up of intestinal bacteria!)

It's even been speculated that these pentose polymers account for the correlation seen in Scandinavia between bulky stools and low colorectal cancer incidence. In Copenhagen, the incidence of colorectal cancer is high, and a small amount of unrefined cereals is eaten. In rural Finland, on the other hand, large amounts of unrefined rye bread are eaten, the stools are bulky and soft, and the incidence of colorectal cancer is quite low. As Burkitt originally proposed, it is likely that dietary fiber reduces the risk of colorectal cancer in several ways: by decreasing the concentration of carcinogens in the stools due to their bulk; by decreasing the amount of time the waste products remain in the bowel; and possibly by changing the proportions or total number of various bacterial species in the bowel, some of which likely produce or destroy carcinogenic metabolites.

In chapter 8, "Along the Alimentary Canal: Overcoming Constipation and its Attendant Ills," you will find complete information about how to maintain adequate fiber in your diet by choosing fresh fruits and vegetables, whole grains, and other foods rich in this important protective substance.

Food Additives

While scientists and public health workers tend to downplay the potential dangers of food additives, it is our contention that these substances represent a significant public health problem. Since the end of World War II, food additives, potential carcinogens, have increased at an unprecedented and alarming rate. New chemicals are introduced and dumped into our foods, usually before they are tested adequately. This is a violation of the general principles of good sense and of toxicology.

The following food additives have all been found to be carcinogenic in one way or another, and must be removed from our food supply. They were clearly listed by Philippe H. Shubik of the University of Nebraska Medical Center in Omaha, and reported in his 1980 paper in *Preventive Medicine*.

Antisprouting chemicals. Maleic hydrazide has been shown to produce tumors when injected into newborn mice. It is used widely by the tobacco industry, and is used to prevent sprouting in various root crops such as potatoes. Be sure to ask your grocer if the potatoes have been sprayed with a root inhibitor. A good test is to put one of your potatoes in a dark area and see if it develops small buds or sprouts. If it does, you can assume that it has *not* been treated with this dangerous chemical.

Another antisprouting chemical which is probably carcinogenic, is called isopropyl-n-phenylcarbamate. When animals' skin was painted with croton oil and then given this chemical, significant levels of cancer were produced. As a result, it was banned in the Netherlands, but nowhere else.

In view of the dangers of such chemicals, the rush toward natural foods is certainly a wise one.

Unhealthy "oral hygiene" products. Chloroform is one of the most noxious of carcinogens. Unfortunately, it is often found as an additive in toothpaste and cough mixtures, which is why "natural" mouth preparations are advised.

In a paper entitled "Mouthwash and Oral Cancer: Carcinogen or Coincidence?" by Dr. Arthur Weaver and co-workers (1979), 200 patients with squamous cell cancer of the head and neck were examined. In this group 11 persons did not use alcoholic beverages and tobacco, but all but one of these 11 patients had used mouthwash many times daily for more than twenty years. Most of them in fact used a type of mouthwash that contained 25-percent alcohol. The authors concluded that mouthwash may be carcinogenic for susceptible persons; the causative agent was the alcohol in the mouthwash.

We subsequently wrote to the senior author and asked, "Is it the alcohol in the mouthwash that incites the cancer, or is it other additives that are present in mouthwashes, such as saccharine?" It is not well-known that most commercial brands of mouthwash, in addition to containing a high percentage of alcohol, also contain colorings, flavorings, and saccharine for sweetening. In response to our letter, we received the following reply from D. B. Smith, D.D.S., chief, Oral and Maxillofacial Surgery at the Veterans Administration Medical Center in Allen Park, Michigan:

> It is quite possible that a number of irritative substances in mouthwashes are culprits and we will be looking for evidence of same. I was unaware that saccharine was a common ingredient of most mouthwashes. In searching for a common denominator we found ethanol and noted more cases in those who used mouthwashes with a higher percentage of alcohol.
>
> Presently we do not plan to isolate ingredients and test their carcinogenicity specifically.

Artificial sweeteners. Certainly there would have been good reason, however, for these investigators to consider the possible dangers of saccharine in mouthwash. Many experiments have demonstrated that saccharine and cyclamates are quite likely carcinogenic. Cyclamate, which was allowed on the market without having been tested properly, is highly suspect. It was classified as a Generally Recognized as Safe material, but had not been tested in any animal system. Saccharine, while generally given a clean bill of health by toxicologists, has not been permitted in foods in Germany since it was first synthesized there in the 1890s!

Artificial food colors. Food colors are another form of additive that should be avoided like the plague. Now, we are not speaking of the natural food colors made from vegetables such as beets or carrots, but of the coal tar dyes that belong on our walls, not in our cells. One of the earlier carcinogenic food colors, Butter Yellow, was well-known for its ability to induce liver tumors in rats, and it was subsequently withdrawn from food. But how many people had innocently consumed Butter Yellow prior to its being withdrawn?

Other forms of Butter Yellow were also potent carcinogens and were in our foods for a while and later withdrawn. Presently we have several colors which are highly suspect, yet continue to be in our foods—primarily Red #2. According to Dr. Shubik, another dye, auramine, "is a compound whose manufacture causes cancer in man which seems to result from an as yet unidentified impurity" (Shubik 1980).

Asbestos in alcoholic beverages. Another contaminant to consider in the cancer question is asbestos, which is widely used in the food industry. For one, it is used as part of the filters in beer making, and in the manufacture of various alcoholic drinks. Surprisingly, Italian vermouth contains one of the highest asbestos contents due to a quirk in its manufacture. Asbestos is *known* to incite cancer and unfortunately is widespread in the environment.

Nitrites in smoked foods. There is no question, when you look at the epidemiology in various parts of the world, that people who consume large amounts of smoked food have higher rates of cancer. In the Baltic states and in Iceland, where smoked fish is consumed, people seem to suffer all too often from one form of cancer or another.

But the technology does exist for eliminating the nitrites and other harmful chemicals that result from the smoking of fish and meats. For example, condensed smoke and liquid smokes can be used as flavoring agents to produce a substitute, and by doing so most of the dangerous polycyclic hydrocarbons could be removed.

Natural foods, with supplementation, safest. We might summarize this rather alarming survey of cancer causation by stating, simply use common sense. Eat foods that have not been packaged or processed to any great extent. Avoid all foods that contain additives, because there are certainly fresh substitutes available. Be sure to take adequate amounts of all the protective vitamins and minerals, particularly vitamin A, vitamin C, vitamin E, and the antioxidant mineral selenium. (See chapter 12 for a guide to proper dosages.) And, if you insist on having breakfast meats such as bacon or ham with your eggs in the morning, be sure to precede this with a glass of fresh-squeezed orange juice or a good dose of vitamin C (which will neutralize some of the nitrites into relatively harmless substances).

Foods Protective Against Cancer

Having seen which foods and food substances may *cause* cancer, we will now look at those foods which can *protect* us from this dread illness.

Certain vegetables, mainly those of the cruciferous variety such as broccoli, turnips, cabbage, cauliflower, and brussels sprouts, have been postulated to protect us against cancer of the colon and possibly other cancers by Graham and Mettlin (1979). These scientists speculate that the indoles contained in these vegetables induce the activity of arylhydrocarbon hydroxylase in the epithelial tissue of the intestine. This compound seems to interfere somehow with the development of carcinogenic compounds. In another study, Graham et al. (1978) found consistent though minimal reductions in the risk of developing cancer with a regular diet of these vegetables; they also referred to earlier studies which point to the same effect. In a case-control study in Japan, Haenszel et al. (1980) have seen a correlation between the incidence of cancer and the amount of cruciferous vegetables eaten. Other workers have found that bladder cancer patients seem to have eaten this type of vegetables less frequently than controls.

Epidemiologists who have studied the diet histories of stomach cancer patients and *high-risk groups* of people, have found that fresh vegetables as well as fresh fruits have consistently been found *lacking* in the diets of the cancer patients, while *starch* has been found to be eaten in *excess*. A frequently advanced hypothesis is that the vegetables and fruits provide vitamin C, vitamin A, and other antioxidants, which protect against the formation of nitrosamine, a potent carcinogen.

Other foods reported by Rawson (1980) that have been found to prevent cancer by detoxifying certain carcinogens, are alfalfa (increases the activity of the antioxidant benzopyrene hydroxylase); soybeans; high-fiber foods; and the vitamin A-rich fruits and vegetables such as carrots, apricots, and others which you will find listed in Table A.1 in the Appendix.

Note how a fiber-rich diet composed of fruits, vegetables, and whole grains is dense with protective nutrients. As the book develops, the same dietary theme will appear repeatedly.

Rate Your Protective Factors Against Cancer

Hopefully, this chapter has shown you how you can replace your fears of cancer with a positive approach to dietary prevention. By choosing the right foods and supplements, we *can* reduce our cancer risk. Now let's see how you presently rate on your building block for cancer prevention.

Building Block #2:

"Eluding the Big C:"
Your Protective Factors Against Cancer

Takes vitamins E & C, & selenium (See p. 37) 10 points	Eats fiber-rich foods (See p. 39) 9 points	Diet is low-fat (no more than 30%) (See p. 36) 8 points
Does not smoke (See p. 33) 7 points	Eats broccoli, cabbage, etc. (See p. 44) 6 points	Takes vitamin A (See p. 39) (Appendix 1, p. 214) 5 points
Avoids nitrites, nitrates, & erythrobates in packaged meat & fish (See p. 35) 4 points	Reads labels to avoid additives (See p. 41) 3 points	Avoids barbecued foods (See p. 34) 2 points

Total the points for your present protective factors.

Your Score Block #2 _____

To page 66

for your next building block

3

IF SUGAR IS SO SWEET, WHY AM I SO BLUE?

Diabetes: Its Prevention and Control

A Deadly Nutritional Disorder

Diabetes mellitus, one of the most common diseases associated with aging, is in the truest sense of the term, a *nutritional disease*. Not only are the onset and incidence of diabetes in adults linked to dietary factors, but the disease itself consists of an inability of the body to utilize the glucose that is supposed to fuel the energy reactions in the cells. Obviously there is something amiss from a nutritional standpoint when our very food acts as a poison!

Diabetes has been with us throughout recorded history. The Ebers Papyrus, written some thirty-five hundred years ago, contains a description of the clinical symptoms of diabetes. More recently, the incidence of the disease has been increasing worldwide at an alarming rate, particularly during the present century and is a major health problem in most developed countries.

At the turn of the century diabetes was only the twenty-seventh highest cause of death in this country, while today it is perhaps the third most frequent underlying cause of death, after heart disease and cancer. It is estimated that as many as ten million people in the United States have diabetes, or five percent of the population. With diabetes still on the increase, it is estimated that at the present rate an American born today and living to the age of seventy, would have a one in five chance of developing the disease (Friedman 1980).

Indeed, diabetes is so widespread today that it is considered almost "normal" for elderly people to have elevated blood sugar levels! Until we learn that what is *common* is not necessarily *normal*, we are going to be caught in an escalating pattern of chronic illness among the older members of our population.

Diabetes takes its toll throughout the body. Besides leading to premature death through its damaging effect on the vascular system, diabetes is the major cause of blindness in middle-aged Americans, and it is an underlying factor in many of the amputations necessitated by gangrene.

The sad thing is that much of this illness and suffering is unnecessary, because most diabetes is preventable, and even curable. And the treatment for most cases of diabetes is simple: diet and weight control. If we ever needed a good reason to maintain adequate nutrition and avoid being overweight, the threat of diabetes and its deadly complications should be sufficient motivation.

How Diabetes Does its Damage

There are many forms of diabetes, with many associated symptoms and varying degrees of severity. But the common characteristic of all diabetics, young and old, mild or severe, is their inability to utilize glucose properly in their systems.

In normal individuals, when food is eaten, the carbohydrates (and, to a lesser extent, the proteins and fats) are converted into glucose, the sugar that provides the fuel for the energy reactions within the cells. The level of glucose in the blood must remain within a fairly narrow "normal range," and so the blood leaving the digestive tract with its load of glucose goes first to the liver rather than circulating throughout the body. In response to the increase in blood sugar following the ingestion of food, the islands of Langerhans, specialized, microscopic structures within the pancreas, secrete the hormone insulin, which is also delivered by the bloodstream directly to the liver. In the liver the glucose is converted, under the influence of insulin, into the starch glycogen, which is stored for future use as an energy reserve. When the liver has stored all the glycogen it can, the excess glucose is converted to fat and stored in the body's adipose tissues. By the time the blood leaves the liver, then, the blood sugar is at a proper concentration. The insulin that is left over from the conversion of glucose into glycogen in the liver also enters the bloodstream, where it enables the body's cells to use the circulating glucose in combustion reactions.

When the pancreas is not able to produce enough insulin, or when the body is not able to use the insulin that is produced, the glucose accumulates in the blood. Some of the glucose is secreted through the kidneys and leaves the body in the urine. Thus, diabetics often have sugar present in the urine. The excess sugar in the blood has many damaging effects, both direct and indirect. There is evidence that the high sugar level in the blood causes direct damage to the kidneys, the nerves, and the eyes. Through the disruption of fat metabolism diabetes does great indirect damage to the circulatory system.

Major Forms of Diabetes

Insulin-dependent diabetes. There are two major forms of diabetes. The first, known as insulin-dependent diabetes, often has its onset in childhood. For this reason it has also been called *juvenile-onset diabetes*, a somewhat misleading term, since the insulin-dependent form of the disease occurs in adults as well. Insulin-dependent diabetes generally begins quite suddenly and progresses rapidly, becoming relatively severe. The insulin-dependent diabetic, once the disease has developed fully, produces little or no insulin and hence is unable to metabolize sugar properly, and must take insulin by injection.

In addition, insulin-dependent diabetics have a tendency to develop ketosis, a condition arising from the incomplete breakdown of fats. Fats cannot be properly metabolized by the body unless glucose is being "burned." In diabetics, due to the lack of insulin, the combustion of glucose cannot take place, and as a result, the fats are only partially broken down, leading to the accumulation of acetone and diacetic acid in the bloodstream, and the depletion of the blood's alkaline stores by the acid. The resulting condition, known as acidosis or ketoacidosis, can be extremely dangerous, progressing from drowsiness to stupor, coma, and finally death. Before the discovery of insulin by Banting, sufferers from this form of diabetes were generally doomed to short lives, dying of diabetic coma. Today the lifelong use of insulin allows the insulin-dependent diabetic to lead a relatively normal life. Although this form of diabetes is still not curable, it is generally manageable with a combination of insulin injections and a carefully controlled diet.

Insulin-dependent diabetes accounts for about ten percent of all diabetes cases.

Noninsulin dependent diabetes. The second, much more common form of diabetes, is known as noninsulin dependent diabetes or maturity-onset diabetes. This form of the disease is usually milder than the insulin-dependent form. It generally comes on in middle or late life and is characterized by a relative deficiency of insulin rather than a complete or near-total absence of the hormone. The pancreas still produces insulin, but not in sufficient quantity; or the diabetic's body does not respond properly to its own insulin. The maturity-onset form of diabetes can generally be kept under control—and even cured—through careful management of diet combined with exercise. In some cases oral medications are also required to maintain control. Noninsulin dependent diabetics are generally not subject to ketoacidosis, except when under unusual stress.

Is diabetes hereditary? It was recognized as long ago as the seventeenth century that there is a hereditary element in diabetes. Even though diabetes does clearly run in families, other factors are also very important in determining who will actually develop the disease. This has been borne out by studies of identical twins. When one member of a twin pair develops diabetes before the age of 40 (that is, "juvenile-onset" diabetes), in only 50 percent of the cases will the other twin also develop the disease. When one twin develops diabetes *after* the age of 40, however, the other twin will also develop the disease in 92 percent of the cases (Friedman 1980, p. 978). It is highly likely that dietary factors, and (as we will see) the tendency to obesity, are more important determinants than heredity alone. If you have a strong family history of diabetes, that should serve as a serious warning to be even more careful to avoid the risk factors that increase the likelihood of your developing the disease.

How Diabetes Is Diagnosed

Maturity-onset diabetes often presents no overt symptoms, and diagnosis will only be made when an elevated blood sugar is noted on routine laboratory testing or when sugar is detected in the urine. The most certain test for diabetes is the glucose tolerance test. After a period of preparation with restricted diet and avoidance of certain substances including caffeine and nicotine, the patient is given a syrupy glucose drink. Blood samples are then taken at intervals over several hours. If the blood sugar is abnormally elevated in response to this "glucose load," the patient has diabetes. A six-hour version of the glucose tolerance test is used to diagnose the related disorder of hypoglycemia, which is characterized by an abnormal *drop* in blood glucose level at some point following the administration of glucose, indicating an overreaction to the glucose load, with excessive production of insulin. (See our discussion of hypoglycemia beginning on page 62.)

Diet as a Causative Factor in Diabetes

As with so many of the "diseases of civilization" that afflict people of middle age and above in Western societies, diabetes has been noted to increase markedly whenever a society switches from a primitive diet to a more Westernized diet high in refined carbohydrates, low in fiber, and high in fats. In a classic study of Yemenite Jews who moved to Israel, Brunner and co-workers showed the influence of dietary change on diabetes incidence. Before moving to Israel, the Yemenites had been geographically isolated from the influences of modern civilization. Upon first moving to Israel, they were found to have a very low incidence of diabetes, only .05 percent. However, Yemenite Jews who had been living in Israel for more than ten years had an incidence of diabetes of .55 percent—a tenfold increase over the incidence in their newly arrived countrymen (Caster 1976).

One of the most significant changes in the American diet during the present century has been the shocking increase in our consumption of refined sugar. The average American now consumes some 120 pounds of refined sugar per year—much of it as "hidden" sugar in prepared or packaged foods. This increased consumption of sugar is having a disastrous effect on the body's ability to handle this substance properly.

Other nutrients also have a harmful effect on glucose tolerance. Caproic acid, present in butterfat and coconut oil, as well as some of the amino acids derived from it—norleucine, leucine, methionine, glutamate, and norvaline—have been found to produce impaired glucose tolerance when fed to rats. Among the commonly available foods that contain various caproic-acid-related substances are corn grits and chicken skin. When these foods were fed to rats they developed elevated blood sugar. Such foods are characteristic of the "poverty diet" of poor blacks in the United States, who rely on grits, greens, and fatback as staples. It is possible that these specific dietary factors may be partly responsible for the extremely high incidence of diabetes among American blacks (Caster 1976).

Obesity and Diabetes

If any one factor can be considered the major culprit in the development of diabetes and in its increased incidence during this century, it is obesity. The changes that have occurred in the composition of the Western diet are inextricably bound up with an accompanying increase in obesity. The same pattern holds true in all modern postindustrial societies. In a worldwide survey, West and Kalbfleisch found that increased economic status, increased sugar, fat, and protein consumption, increased obesity, and decreased glucose tolerance, all went hand in hand (Friedman 1980, p. 984). Of the estimated ten million diabetics in the United States today, *nine million* of these cases are believed to be obesity-induced (Friedman 1980)!

Just as obesity is more common and more severe with increasing age in our society, so does the incidence and degree of diabetes increase with age. Eighty percent of the cases of diabetes in this country are of the obese, adult-onset type, and *ninety percent of all known diabetics were overweight at the time their diabetes was discovered*. (Some diabetics succeed in losing weight after their disease is diagnosed.) In societies where obesity is uncommon, so is diabetes; where obesity has been common for twenty years or more, diabetes is also common. From Micronesia to Zululand, from Bengalis to Australian aborigines, the message is the same: When obesity becomes epidemic, usually as a result of a change to the refined foods of the Western diet, diabetes also becomes epidemic.

Animal studies also show that weight control prevents diabetes. In experiments with hamsters, it was observed that even when the animals were selectively bred to be diabetes-prone, caloric restriction alone could prevent or delay the onset of diabetes and prevent premature death and pathological complications of the disease. The diabetes-prone, or "prediabetic," hamsters, when fed as much as they desired, tended to eat more than nonprediabetic control animals (Gerritson 1976).

There have not been any comparable studies of the effects of caloric restriction in prediabetic humans, mainly because it is so difficult to control overeating patterns in people, even when they know that they are at high risk for diabetes. But circumstantial evidence—such as the decreased incidence of new cases of diabetes in European countries during wartime, when caloric intake was restricted—seems to point to a similar pattern in humans.

The evidence is clear: The single most important precipitating factor in the vast majority of cases of maturity-onset diabetes is excessive caloric intake, and the obesity that results. For each twenty percent of excess body weight, the chances of developing diabetes are doubled.

Weight loss reduces diabetic symptoms. Not only can weight control prevent diabetes, but it can also cure it. When obese diabetics of the maturity-onset type lose weight and control their caloric intake, their blood sugar levels are often reduced and their need for insulin or other medications is decreased or eliminated!

Being overweight by itself apparently contributes to disturbances in blood sugar levels. It has been shown that obese people are relatively insensitive to their own insulin. Their body cells contain fewer "insulin receptors" to take insulin from the blood and metabolize glucose within the cell. Obese people therefore need to produce more insulin, and they have high basal levels of fasting insulin in their blood. (Incidentally, high levels of fasting insulin are among the most predictive "risk factors" for the development of coronary heart disease.) Their chronically overworked pancreatic cells may break down progressively, until they finally stop producing insulin entirely.

Treating Diabetes with Diet

Although insulin-dependent diabetics will not be able to throw away their insulin syringes simply by eating carefully controlled diets, they may be able to reduce their insulin dosage. But in that vast majority of diabetics of the noninsulin-dependent or maturity-onset type, diabetes is now considered in many cases to be curable. Particularly in recently diagnosed cases of obesity-related diabetes, a return to normal weight is usually able to completely reverse the disease process. Even in diabetics of long-standing, weight loss will generally reduce the severity of the disease to a considerable extent. Diet is thus the *first and most important* element in the treatment of the newly diagnosed noninsulin-dependent diabetic.

Before the discovery of insulin in 1921, the only treatment available to keep juvenile-onset diabetics alive was dietary. The prescribed diet was high in fats and proteins, with carbohydrates virtually eliminated since they tended to elevate blood sugar. This so-called ketogenic diet results in the production of ketone bodies from fats broken down to supply energy, when dietary carbohydrates are missing. Some of the recent reducing diets are a return to the ketogenic principle, which bypasses the use of carbohydrates to provide energy and forces the body to use up its stores of fat instead.

When insulin injections and oral medications became available for diabetic control, it became possible to liberalize the carbohydrate allowances of the diabetic diet, so that today a more varied combination of nutrients is favored.

Carbohydrates. Currently most experts recommend a low-fat, high-carbohydrate diet that favors complex carbohydrates over refined sugars and white flour. Each diabetic's diet must be individualized, taking into consideration the patient's weight, level of activity, other medical problems if any, food likes and dislikes, and ethnic dietary preferences. In general, however, a diabetic diet might contain from 40 percent to as much as 60 percent of the calories in the form of carbohydrates. It is very important that the carbohydrate foods be rich in nutritional value, avoiding the empty calories of refined sugars and starches, and stressing whole grains and fresh fruits and vegetables. It is noteworthy that in Asia diabetics usually eat high-carbohydrate diets, up to 70 percent, and their diabetes is usually very mild. The incidence of coronary atherosclerosis is also very low in Asian populations, thanks in part to the low-fat, high-carbohydrate diet.

Complex-carbohydrate foods have the additional benefit of providing high *fiber* content in the diet. We will show in chapter 8 how fiber protects against constipation and related disorders. In addition, fiber seems to have specific benefits in diabetes. It lowers blood sugar, de-

creases the excretion of sugar in the urine, and reduces
the diabetic's need for insulin. Anderson (1981) notes that
water-retaining fibers such as pectin and guar, are particularly effective in smoothing out the peaks and valleys of
the blood glucose curve. He reports as follows on the
results of high-carbohydrate (55–60 percent) diets for
diabetics, in which 75 percent of the carbohydrates are in
the complex form:

> High-carbohydrate, high-fiber diets have allowed
> us to reduce insulin doses in every patient we have
> treated. For example, 20 lean patients were receiving
> an average of 27 units of insulin/day on their standard
> diets. With the high-carbohydrate, high-fiber diets,
> their average insulin doses dropped to 7 units/day. We
> were eventually able to discontinue insulin therapy in
> 15 of these 20 patients. These reductions in insulin
> dose were not related to weight loss since the patients
> maintained the same lean weight.
>
>   (Anderson 1981, pp. 1–2)

Careful planning of the diabetic diet must taken into
consideration the metabolic differences between various
starches and sugars. It may be of value to specify the
approximate amounts of various carbohydrates in order to
avoid overworking the body's sugar-processing mechanisms
and producing undesirable side effects such as hypoglycemia.

Fructose, which is half of the sucrose molecule, or
refined sugar, has become increasingly popular recently.
Nearly twice as sweet as sucrose, fructose is being used
increasingly in "diet drinks" and "health foods." Because it
is sweeter than ordinary sugar, the reasoning goes, less
fructose is required for the same taste, and so theoretically,
it produces less overall hormonal stress than sucrose.
Unfortunately, however, although fructose does not cause
as great a rise in blood glucose concentration as do sucrose
or glucose, it can increase serum triglycerides, just as
these other simple sugars can.

Fat. The amount and kind of fat must be carefully
controlled in the diabetic diet. The American Diabetic
Association's Committee on Food and Nutrition, in its
1979 guidelines, specified that 30–38 percent of the total

calories should be fat, with saturated fats constituting less than 10 percent of the calories, polyunsaturated fats constituting another 10 percent, and the remainder being monounsaturated fats.

Diabetics are particularly prone to atherosclerosis and its deadly effects such as coronary heart disease, high blood pressure, and occlusive vascular disease. In fact, the primary cause of death in diabetics is the vascular disease associated with the diabetic condition. Because diabetics are more likely than nondiabetics to have elevated blood cholesterol and triglycerides (two indicators of high risk for atherosclerotic disease), it is very important to regulate the diet to keep these blood lipids under control. Although the evidence is still equivocal, it appears that one significant factor in elevated blood lipid levels is high levels of saturated fats (and perhaps cholesterol) in the diet. We must warn, however, that there is also danger in the overconsumption of polyunsaturated fats, for there is now good evidence that polyunsaturates are a source of harmful free radical reactions that may be an underlying cause of cancer and other "diseases of aging." So you must strike a balance by eating a variety of fats, moderately.

Protein. If you are a diabetic, 12–20 percent of your total calories should be protein. Some dietary protein and protein in body cells can be transformed into glucose, leading to a rise in blood sugar. However, since the conversion of protein into glucose is relatively slow, protein foods help to maintain stable blood sugar levels over several hours' time. Poorly controlled diabetes may lead to the depletion of essential protein in body tissues, as well as the accelerated breakdown of dietary proteins. When excessive protein is being converted into glucose in the diabetic's body, it may be necessary to *increase* protein intake in order to protect against damage to vital tissues. Other situations where increased protein may be required are in pregnancy, infection, or some chronic illnesses. In the case of liver or kidney failure, on the other hand, protein intake may need to be reduced to avoid overworking the damaged organ.

Alcohol. Wine was used as an empirical treatment of diabetes some 1600 years before the discovery of insulin.

Although alcohol produces hypoglycemia, or a drop in blood sugar, in some individuals, obese people and diabetics seem to be generally resistant to this effect. Thus there is no metabolic reason why diabetics cannot drink alcohol, and in fact, since it is metabolized without requiring insulin, it can be a relatively harmless adjunct to diabetic therapy, offering you a mild relaxant effect of real psychological benefit.

Wine is actually recommended in the diabetic diet for these reasons, but a few warnings must be kept in mind. First of all, alcohol does contain calories. The higher the alcohol content of a drink, the higher is its calorie count. For this reason it is wise to stick with dry wine and to avoid the higher-calorie, higher-proof liquors. Of course, sweetened mixers add even more calories in a mixed drink and should be avoided. Beer is just too caloric to be anything but harmful.

A common strategy for diabetics is to substitute a glass of wine for its caloric equivalent of fat in the day's dietary allocation.

Coffee. Caffeine has a complex effect on our metabolism. It stimulates the production of hormones that trigger the conversion of glycogen into glucose in the liver, and then stimulates the pancreas to produce more insulin. All this can add up to a hypoglycemic reaction, or at least an elevation of blood insulin levels. Elevated blood insulin may increase hunger pangs, and therefore is undesirable for anyone who is trying to control his or her weight.

Because of these metabolic effects, it is not a good idea for diabetics to consume coffee, or any other caffeine-containing beverages, for that matter—and that includes black and green teas, and diet colas. Try mild herbal teas instead, such as chamomile or linden, or one of the herbal or cereal-based coffee substitutes.

Calculating the diabetic diet. Especially for insulin-dependent diabetics, careful calculations are required to produce a diet that will prevent marked fluctuations in blood sugar and ketones and avoid the toxic states that characterize the disease, as well as the long-term damage that can be done to the organs through exposure to elevated levels of blood glucose. Expert medical advice is needed in this regard, with regular reassessment of all factors involved.

Diabetics generally learn to plan their day's meal in terms of *exchanges*, or calorically equivalent servings of various classes of nutrients, so that a certain number of fat exchanges, protein exchanges, and carbohydrate exchanges are allowed during the day. If you are an insulin-dependent diabetic you may also need to take multiple small feedings rather than eat three large meals a day, in order to avoid excessive rises in blood sugar levels. If you miss a usual meal, you may need to replace the carbohydrates with a sweet drink in order to avoid an insulin reaction.

Relearning eating habits. At least as important as calculations of exchanges is the development of a whole new set of habits and attitudes toward eating. This goes for all diabetics, and particularly for the large proportion who are overweight. Whereas nondiabetic Americans may manage to get by for years with their weight yo-yoing up and down, for the obese diabetic, weight control can be literally a matter of life and death. If your doctor or dietitian doesn't place the highest possible emphasis on controlling weight and caloric intake, perhaps you should look for professional help elsewhere for your diabetic control. Counseling can be a very useful adjunct to diet therapy, in order to maintain the highest possible level of motivation. Special techniques for altering eating patterns, such as behavior modification therapy, may be useful for diabetic patients who have difficulty sticking to their diets.

Within limits, your diabetic diet should reflect your normal ethnic food preferences, since these will fit in with your family's life-style. However, some modern "ethnic" diets in this country are based on "poverty budgets" and are high in refined carbohydrates and fats—which may be cheaper to buy at the market but take a much heavier toll on health, particularly of the diabetic patient. The diabetic diet may be a little more expensive to prepare than these low-budget diets. But whole grains and fresh fruits and vegetables bought in season, are very reasonable in price. These foods should be a staple part of your daily food intake. Sweets, white bread, white rice, white spaghetti, sodas, and junk foods, are more expensive in the long run because they are nutritionally "empty," providing little but calories for their cost.

Traveling and dining out need not present insurmountable obstacles either. Once you are familiar with your diet plan it will be possible for you to make selections from a restaurant menu with confidence. Remember that restaurant portions may be larger than allowed on your diet, so don't hesitate to leave food uneaten. Ask for sauces and dressings to be served on the side, or not at all; and remove batters from fried foods before eating them. Particularly in the fast-food chains, servings and preparation methods are highly standardized, and the caloric and nutritional content of many chains' menus have been extensively analyzed and documented. Once you know what's between those hamburger buns, you can choose intelligently and avoid overly greasy or calorie-laden foods.

When you're invited to dinner at the home of friends, don't hesitate to ask what they'll be serving and at what time. If dinner will be later than the accustomed time, the insulin-dependent diabetic may need to eat a light snack (such as rice crackers) before leaving home in order to prevent an insulin reaction. It's a good idea also to bring along a piece of fresh fruit for dessert that can be enjoyed without making a "scene."

Exercise. In the treatment of all diabetes, exercise is an important accompaniment to careful dietary control. Not only does exercise help to use up calories, but improving your physical conditioning also contributes to more efficient functioning of the insulin-producing cells of the pancreas. If you haven't been engaging in regular exercise, it's essential that you have a medical checkup and some professional guidance in setting up an exercise program. Particularly in the case of the complications that may accompany diabetes, such as high blood pressure and vascular disease, a sudden, unaccustomed strain on the cardiovascular system can have serious, potentially lethal consequences. In the next chapter we will discuss the dietary supplements that will help support your exercise program.

Dietary Supplements in Diabetes

The diabetic's requirements for vitamins and minerals are generally the same as they are for nondiabetics, with a few important exceptions where additional supplementation may be wise. Of course, for anyone on a reducing diet, as many diabetics are, vitamin supplementation is an absolute necessity. Any diet that contains 1,000 calories or less per day must definitely be supplemented with vitamins and minerals. Here a good multiple-vitamin and mineral capsule would be the first line of defense against deficiency states.

Vitamin A. Diabetics may have an impaired ability to manufacture vitamin A from carotene in the diet. Among other functions, vitamin A is essential to ensure adequate production of cortisone, which balances the effects of insulin. The diabetic diet should be rich in foods containing vitamin A, including carrots, apricots, liver, eggs, whole milk, and cheese (within caloric and fat limits), but additional supplementation may be called for, especially during periods of illness or stress. The usual therapeutic range is 10,000–20,000 International Units daily. (See chapter 12 for a guide to proper dosages.)

Vitamin C. There is some evidence that high doses of vitamin C can reduce insulin requirements in "juvenile-onset" diabetics. One of the many functions of this important vitamin is to help regulate the utilization of sugar. Fresh fruits and vegetables should provide considerable vitamin C, but since an individual's needs may far exceed the presently defined minimum daily requirement, this is another vitamin that may need to be supplemented. Therapeutic dosages of vitamin C range from 500 milligrams to 5,000 milligrams daily.

Vitamin B complex. Among the B vitamins that may need to be supplemented, perhaps in the form of B complex, are folic acid and B_6. These vitamins are depleted by certain medications, such as oral contraceptives; check with your physician to see if your needs are increased by any drugs you are taking. Table 10.1 in chapter 10 lists some common prescription drugs and the nutrients that may need to be supplemented when they are used.

Minerals. Dairy products will help to supply your calcium needs. If you are restricting your caloric intake, low-fat milk or low-fat yogurt are good calcium sources. Cottage cheese, however, is *low* in calcium owing to the processing it undergoes. Other excellent sources of calcium are soft fish bones (as in herring, sardines, or salmon), and dark green leafy vegetables. Dried figs, broccoli, baked beans, and dried legumes are all good calcium sources as well.

Iron is another mineral that is often deficient in the diet, and may need to be supplemented. Diabetics who are under poor control, or who use large quantities of insulin, may also have imbalances in electrolytes, particularly potassium. Sodium and potassium intake may need to be carefully regulated when there is accompanying disease of the kidneys, the liver, or the cardiovascular system. Good sources of potassium are dates, figs, potatoes, peaches, apricots, bananas, raisins, peanuts (*unsalted*), and seafood.

Chromium and the glucose tolerance factor. A recently identified dietary factor, consisting of trivalent chromium and three amino acids, has been found to be essential in glucose tolerance in rats, and may be essential for humans as well. Chromium levels are often depleted in diabetics. One reason a high-fiber diet may help to lower blood glucose is that fiber-rich foods are also rich in chromium and other important nutrients.

In its bound form, chromium activates insulin, helping to convert sugar into usable glycogen or fatty acids. Foods such as yeast, mushrooms, wheat germ, oysters, American cheese, and whole wheat bread, contain some glucose tolerance factor, or GTF, but by far the richest source is brewer's yeast. There is now a new form of brewer's yeast called GTF yeast in which the GTF is even more concentrated, and it can be conveniently mixed into your favorite blender-made drink.

Hypoglycemia: Pseudo-Diabetes

The other side of the coin of impaired carbohydrate metabolism is reactive hypoglycemia, or low blood sugar.

While many medical authorities remain skeptical as to how widespread this condition is, there can be little doubt that some hypoglycemics have been mistakenly diagnosed as diabetic and have received no help—and perhaps some harm—from the usual diabetic treatment. (Hypoglycemia has been mistaken for many other diseases as well—from mental retardation to rheumatoid arthritis!)

It was Dr. Seale Harris who first described hypoglycemia in an article in the *Journal of the American Medical Association* back in 1924. Dr. Harris noticed that some nondiabetic individuals manifested the same kinds of symptoms that diabetics experienced when they took too large a dose of insulin and went into insulin shock: faintness, hunger, palpitations, cold sweat, and other disturbances. Dr. Harris reasoned that these people were suffering from hyperinsulinism, an excessive secretion of insulin by the pancreas, which resulted in a drop in blood sugar below normal levels and led to the complex of symptoms he observed.

According to Carlton Fredericks, Ph.D., in his excellent book *Low Blood Sugar and You* (1969), the following symptoms were all reported by hypoglycemic patients treated by Dr. Stephen Gyland, another pioneer in the field:

> nervousness, irritability, exhaustion, faintness, dizziness, tremor, cold sweats, weak spells, depression, vertigo, drowsiness, headaches, digestive disturbances, forgetfulness, insomnia, constant worrying, mental confusion, internal trembling, heart palpitation, muscular pain, numbness, asocial, antisocial, or unsocial behavior, indecisiveness, crying spells, loss of sex drive in females, allergies, incoordination, leg cramps, poor concentration, blurred vision, twitching and jerking of muscles, itching and crawling sensations on the skin, gasping for breath, smothering spells, staggering, sighing and yawning, male impotence, unconsciousness, night terrors, nightmares, rheumatoid arthritis, phobias, neurodermatitis, suicidal intent, nervous breakdown, convulsions.

With such a wide range of manifestations, it is no wonder that hypoglycemia has been scoffed at and called

the nonillness of the decade! But for people who are
caught on the seesaw of rising and falling blood sugar
levels, these symptoms can be a very serious matter indeed.
In a society that consumes such vast quantities of refined
sugars and starches, it's understandable that many people
have lost the ability to metabolize carbohydrates properly.

Reactive hypoglycemia is diagnosed by a six-hour glucose tolerance test. Whereas a true diabetic will show an
elevated blood sugar level throughout this test, the hypoglycemic will first show a rise in blood sugar in response to
the glucose load, and then during the last couple of hours
the blood sugar will drop *below* the fasting level. Thus,
the hypoglycemic's symptoms of anxiety, hunger, faintness,
and so on, develop four hours or so after eating, at the
point when the blood sugar drops below normal owing to
the oversecretion of insulin in response to the meal.

Dr. Fredericks describes a much quicker test, and he
claims it is amazingly accurate:

> Basically, the Goodman test calls for a determination
> of the fasting blood sugar level before breakfast. The
> patient is then instructed to eat his normal breakfast,
> and the test is repeated 45 minutes to one hour later.
> If the blood sugar at that time has not risen 50 percent
> or more above the fasting level, the patient is hypo-
> glycemic, and this is true even though the initial and
> the second readings both fall within "normal range."
> This may be compared with the long test, in which
> many blood sugar levels are determined over a six-
> hour period after sugar has been fed as a challenge to
> the pancreas.
>
> (Fredericks 1969, p. 111)

Diet to correct hypoglycemia. In the final analysis,
the best test for reactive hypoglycemia is a trial of the
therapeutic diet. If, when you follow the diet we will now
describe, your symptoms disappear, it is a pretty safe bet
that you were suffering from low blood sugar.

The objective of the diet is to prevent rapid rises in
blood sugar and blood insulin, to avoid the rebounding
drop in blood sugar. To keep blood sugar at as steady a
level as possible, eat protein-rich foods such as lean meat,

fish, and skinned poultry and dairy products. Avoid fried food since it is relatively indigestible. Vegetables may include broccoli, chard, cabbage, cucumbers, cauliflower, eggplant, spinach, lettuce, tomato, string beans, and kale. Fruits should be eaten fresh or frozen, without sugar syrups and, if dried, without sugar added. Allowable fruits include apples, berries, melons, pears, and peaches. Oranges and grapefruit may be eaten, but only in moderation. You may eat unrefined carbohydrates in unlimited quantities—whole grains, potatoes, sweet potatoes, lentils, and legumes. These complex carbohydrates are metabolized slowly and help to maintain blood sugar at a stable level.

Strictly forbidden for the hypoglycemic are all foods containing sugar—and that means watching out for the hidden sugars in ketchup, sauces, gravies, and many other processed foods. Also to be avoided are all soft drinks, including diet soft drinks, any fruit drinks that contain sugar sweetener, and any caffeine-containing beverages, including coffee, black tea, colas, and cocoa drinks. Alcoholic beverages, unfortunately, are also on the forbidden list.

The recommended foods should be distributed over six small meals a day, rather than the usual three large meals. This strategy is a very important factor in stabilizing blood sugar.

You may wonder whether you will need to stick to this diet for the rest of your life. After perhaps six months, under careful professional guidance, you may be able to resume eating some of the foods you have been avoiding, but this must be done very cautiously or you will find yourself back on the seesaw again.

Rate Your Protective Factors for Diabetes

The principles of dietary treatment of diabetes also make good sense as preventive measures. Let's take a look at your building block and see how you can protect yourself against this very common disease of midlife and beyond.

Building Block #3:

"If Sugar Is so Sweet, Why Am I so Blue?"
Your Protective Factors Against Diabetes

Keeps weight within 10% of ideal (See p. 53) 10 points	Eats whole, high-fiber foods (40–60% of diet) (See p. 55) 9 points	Fat in diet 30% or less (See p. 56) 8 points
Exercises regularly (See p. 60) 7 points	Avoids caffeine (See p. 58) 6 points	Eats fruits in place of sweet desserts (See p. 55) 5 points
Gets "glucose tolerance factor" in food or supplement (See p.62) 4 points	Takes vitamins A (10,000–20,000 IU) & B complex (See p. 61) 3 points	Drinks a little wine (See p. 57) 2 points

Total the points for your present protective factors.

Your Score
Block #3 _____

To page 77

for your next building block

4

VITAMIN E AND THE AGING JOCK:

Nutrients to Support Your Exercise Program

Exercise "Supplements" for the Sedentary

We can hardly expect all Americans to give up their desk jobs and return to tilling the fields. To compensate for our overly sedentary style of living, many people have taken up vigorous exercise—running, swimming, and other such activities—that provide needed cardiorespiratory conditioning. Exercise physiologists have determined that as little as twenty minutes of sustained, vigorous exercise, three times a week, is sufficient to achieve a conditioning effect. Such a program of vigorous exercise can be combined with other activities such as stretching or yoga for flexibility, and some sort of resistance training, in which the body must work against gravity, to achieve strength, vigor, and ease of movement in all parts of the body.

Of course, the simpler, less "jockish" activities, such as taking long walks, dancing, and making love, can be a source of great pleasure at the same time that they help maintain the condition of the body and afford the opportunity for social interaction. For many people these forms of exercise prove ideal.

For those of you who have taken up the new all-American sport of jogging or running, the following article should be of particular interest. Adapted from the original version in *Runner's World* magazine (Weiner and Rothschild 1980), it points out the important connection between your exercise program and vitamin supplementation.

The Vitamin that Likes Oxygen

How nutrition supports endurance. Physical endurance is the key to achievement in many sports. Most researchers agree that athletes need additional energy to keep fit and to compensate for physical exertion and stress. Long-distance runners and other athletes who compete in endurance sports, require vitamin and mineral supplementation, especially vitamin E, which improves the circulation of oxygen in the heart and muscles. For the aging sportsperson, nutrient supplementation can be especially critical.

Aerobic capacity, otherwise known as efficiency of oxygen consumption, must be high enough to prevent muscle fatigue. Fatigue is a result of oxygen starvation in the blood. Numerous studies have proven that vitamin E levels decline as oxygen requirements increase, and are related to fatigue. Vitamin E, combined with aerobic exercise, increases the oxygen-carrying capacity of hemoglobin in the blood, leading to greater dynamic capabilities of the lungs. Since stores of this vitamin are depleted during stress, a case can be made for the need of vitamin E supplements to ensure physical stamina.

Discovery of vitamin E. Vitamin E was first discovered in 1922 by Dr. Herbert Evans and Dr. Kathryn Bishop of the University of California at Berkeley, and labeled "factor X" after it was recognized that this dietary constituent was essential for successful reproduction in animals. By 1925, vitamin E was adopted into the vitamin family, following the system of alphabetic designation of its predecessors.

Sterility was the first condition noted in vitamin E deficiency. Research over the next ten years revealed numerous deficiency states, the most noteworthy being nutritional muscular dystrophy in mammals. In 1936, Dr. Evans first isolated vitamin E from wheat germ oil, which has the highest concentration of the vitamin among all plant foods.

Other rich natural sources of vitamin E are salad oils, fats, seeds (especially almonds and peanuts), and margarine. Some green leafy vegetables contain significant amounts of vitamin E, as do fresh asparagus and mangos. However, processed, packaged, and stored foods may be notoriously deficient in vitamin E activity; 80 percent or more of vitamin E is lost in converting whole wheat to white bread, with freezing of vegetables also causing great losses.

Vitamin E occurs as four different compounds called tocopherols. The name *tocopherol* is derived from the Greek *tokos* (offspring) and *pherein* (to bear). It is no wonder that shortly after its discovery, vitamin E became commonly known as the antisterility factor. Since then, researchers throughout the world have discovered a demonstrated need of vitamin E for proper maintenance and function of skeletal muscle and cardiovascular tone.

Making the most of oxygen. Recently, much attention has been focused on the influence of vitamin E on muscular activity. Numerous claims have been cited on the value of vitamin E in avoiding fatigue. In an address to the Japanese Society for Sports Medicine, Dr. Jyunichiki told a group of physicians that vitamin E facilitates the utilization of oxygen by athletes and reduces the accumulation of lactic acid, a toxic metabolite that causes muscle fatigue. By supplementing their diet with vitamin E, runners and other endurance athletes can extend their collapse point.

While runners race over the marathon course, the blood coursing through their veins often affects the results. Oxygen transport and utilization are two of the most important factors leading to success in a marathon. In competition, good marathon runners are highly efficient and use only fifty-six to sixty milliliters of oxygen per kilogram per minute while maintaining a pace of ten to twelve miles per hour. Trained long-distance runners use up a significantly smaller proportion of their maximum capacity to consume oxygen, thus reducing negative stress and the resulting exhaustion.

When more oxygen is available in the bloodstream, there is less stress on the heart to pump blood through the vessels. Some researchers believe that vitamin E helps promote aerobic pathways, which ensure an adequate supply of oxygen and the ability of the working cells to utilize that oxygen. Proper oxygenation of cerebral blood flow is necessary for mental as well as physical stamina.

Although vitamin E is fat soluble, it is nontoxic, even in extremely high doses. The highest concentrations are found in the pituitary, the master gland of the body, and in the adrenals, which produce the energy-generating hormone, adrenaline. Vitamin E, in addition to iron, folic acid, B_6, B_{12}, C, copper, and protein, is a necessary component in the intricate pathways that ensure the proper function of bone marrow.

How to tell if you are deficient. The most visible sign of vitamin E deficiency is muscular dystrophy. This pernicious nutritional deficiency is comparable to scurvy, the result of vitamin E deficiency, and beriberi, the deficiency state of vitamin B_1. Early signs of vitamin E deficiency include emaciation, skin ulcers, and tremors. Cystic fibrosis, a disease that diminishes the elasticity of the lungs, is also associated with vitamin E deficiency. Muscle degeneration is the most damaging example of vitamin E deficiency.

Only recently have nutritional scientists begun to explore and understand the full significance of vitamin E's function as an antioxidant that protects the structural integrity of the cell membrane. *Antioxidant* is a biochemical term for any substance that prevents the deterioration of cellular materials through the oxidative process, for example, protecting food fats from turning rancid. As an antioxidant, vitamin E also guards against the stresses in vigorous exercise. If you are a long-distance runner, megadoses of vitamin E (1,000 international units (IU) a day) may be valuable in reducing night leg cramps.

Protective nutrients. Among the most significant benefits of vitamin E is its ability to neutralize the formation of nitrosamines from nitrates, and to protect against the cancer-causing effects of lead, mercury, and cadmium. Vitamin E also guards against forms of toxic free radicals, substances that accelerate the aging process. Research scientists at the Linus Pauling Institute of Science and Medicine, have demonstrated the role of the antioxidants vitamin C, vitamin E, and selenium in preventing the proliferation of certain cancer cells.

In a discussion with Dr. Richard Kunin, president of the Orthomolecular Medical Society, we learned of Packer and Slater's recent findings on the interactions of vitamins C and E. These researchers reported the synergistic actions of these vitamins and the recycling of vitamin E at the expense of vitamin C. *The more vitamin C you take, the less vitamin E you need.* Here is another example of the vital role vitamin C plays in the optimal utilization of vitamin E. Vitamin C metabolism is interrelated with the mineral magnesium, to the point where the vitamin is useless without it. Neuromuscular irritability is lessened, proper elimination is promoted, body temperature regulation is influenced, and teeth are strengthened, all by the silvery white metal, magnesium.

We recommend approximately 270 milligrams of magnesium daily, and more if vitamin C is supplemented in the diet, as it should be. The best sources of magnesium are wheat bran, wheat germ, soybeans, brewer's yeast, black walnuts, and roasted peanuts. Other foods rich in this important mineral are brussels sprouts, chard, corn, peas, prunes, raisins, and spinach.

Another promising finding is the therapeutic use of vitamin E in preventing clotting disorders in women using oral contraceptives. As far as men are concerned, vitamin E may enhance the possibility of overcoming infertility and is commonly prescribed to increase sperm count and sperm activity.

Reduction in serum cholesterol is also associated with this vitamin. Recently, research enzymologists discovered that a complex relationship exists between vitamin E and the nutritional stress imposed by the presence of fats in a person's diet, especially polyunsaturated fat. People eating large amounts of vegetable oils, especially those rich in linoleic acid (for example, corn, cottonseed, and soybean) need *more* vitamin E. This is why we recommend unrefined, cold-pressed olive oil. Here is a monosaturated oil (a mix between saturated and polyunsaturated fats) with a great history among Mediterranean people known for their resistance to the diseases of aging.

Another purported benefit of vitamin E is that it improves circulation by keeping the blood density down. When the hematocrit, or red blood cell concentration, is too high, lethargic circulation can result, body cells would be starved of their nutrients, and cellular waste materials would be improperly eliminated. Such degenerative problems as strokes, high blood pressure, and kidney malfunctions can result.

When the fatty acids in the bloodstream oxidize or go rancid, oxygen is lost in the process. By blocking the oxidation of fatty acids, vitamin E releases more oxygen to service the body's tissues and muscles.

Medical anthropologists have reported immunity to athersclerosis among the Masai warriors of East Africa, who herd cattle on foot, and also among the Tarahumara Indians of Mexico, who take part in ceremonial runs. The diets of both groups consist mainly of unrefined vegetable grains high in vitamin E.

In 1972, reports from Swedish researchers indicated that men recovering from heart attacks, who were taking vitamin E supplements as part of their daily diet, had developed prolonged blood-clotting time. The doctors suggested that this positive change might be due to the fact that large daily doses of vitamin E depress the vitamin K-dependent coagulation factor. With a prolonged blood-clotting time, a person's blood flows more freely, helping to prevent a recurrence of heart attacks. Traditionally, doctors use such strong drugs as heparin and dicumarol to produce this effect. However, these drugs often have powerful, negative side effects.

The combination of regular, moderate exercise and vitamin supplementation with a rational diet, offers the greatest protection against the development of heart disease.

E against stress. In urban environments where smog

diminishes air quality, there is an increased need for anti-oxidants such as vitamin C, vitamin E, and selenium. Smog is an environmental stress on the oxygen-carrying potential of the circulatory system. At times, veteran runners collapse before completing marathons in urban areas. Numerous reports have cited the protective effect of vitamin E on the sensitivity of lung tissue to air pollution. The predominant oxidant in the atmosphere is smog. Vitamin E, as an antioxidant, helps to neutralize smog's damaging effects.

Running puts stress on the cardiovascular, respiratory, and neuromuscular systems. In long-distance running, the neuromuscular system, especially the nerves and long muscles of the legs, experiences the greatest stress. Stress is also implicated in decreased longevity. In recent years, vitamin E has been labeled the "antistress factor." Vitamin E facilitates oxygen transport to the blood and is particularly beneficial in competitions taking place in a rarefied atmosphere, such as in Mexico City, site of the 1968 Summer Olympics.

The question of dosage. In 1968, the Food and Nutrition Board of the FDA announced a recommended daily allowance for vitamin E of 30 IU a day. In searching the scientific literature on vitamin E, no state of hypervitaminosis or vitamin toxicity has been reported, even among adults who ingested one gram a day for several months. In 1974, a new subcommittee lowered the requirement to 15 IU—in spite of data showing that vitamin E is essential in protecting the integrity of the blood cells and muscle tissue. In addition to their questionable calculations, the board has also ignored the fact that much vitamin E is lost in food processing and storage and must be replaced by supplementation.

Although overt deficiency states of vitamin E in the United States are rare, nutritionally conscious people are more concerned about *optimal* nutrition than about the minimum level designated by the FDA. If a deficiency state of Vitamin E causes muscle degeneration, then taking the optimal level of this nontoxic vitamin will probably increase an athlete's muscular efficiency.

Government skepticism and empirical enthusiasm. The federal government has allocated millions of dollars for research designed to investigate the scientific claims supporting nutrient therapy. The FDA has traditionally placed tough restrictions on researchers who work with vitamins, demanding evidence from long-term studies only. Yet, the same demands are not always placed on studies that criticize vitamin supplementation. Some research that has refuted the health benefits of vitamins has been based on subjective questionnaires distributed to an unrepresentative population group that lacked control groups and rigorous scientific standards of evaluation.

A recent panel-study by the FDA recommended restrictions on the sale of vitamin and mineral preparations such as brewer's yeast, kelp, wheat germ, and lecithin. The FDA claimed that these natural ingredients did not contribute to the effectiveness of products treating degenerative diseases.

The FDA panel suggested that all ingredients labeled as therapeutic should be dispensed by prescription only. Although prescription sales of vitamins appear remote at this time, if the trend in FDA rulings continues, that is exactly what may occur: The health-conscious consumer will have to pay a doctor for a vitamin prescription and then tack on the increased cost of purchasing vitamins from a pharmacist rather than a food store.

The FDA has pointed to the lack of scientific evidence demonstrating the therapeutic efficacy of vitamin and mineral products as a rationale for recommending removal of the substances from general availability.

The vitamin proponents of the Orthomolecular Medical Society, a worldwide group of doctors who believe in using nutrient therapy—vitamins and minerals—in treating diseases, disagree. While they admit that conclusive evidence of the benefits of vitamins has not been established, they also feel that the public should be educated and encouraged to avail themselves of the potential benefits of nutritional therapy.

Doctors who use nutrients as pharmacological tools have had similar success in treating degenerative diseases as physicians who employ conventional drugs, often without the serious side effects these drugs have been known to cause.

However, the proponents of *orthomolecular treatment* (a term coined by Linus Pauling to describe the optimal concentration of nutrients present in the body) do not believe in self-medication. Vitamins in high dosages can be potentially damaging if users don't know what they are doing.

Cautions! Dr. William Cathcart III, an orthopedic surgeon who has worked in sports medicine and been involved in research with Linus Pauling, cautions:

> People who take vitamin E, especially heart patients and diabetics, should do so only under proper medical advice. Because vitamin E is a strong heart stimulant, high doses can increase the blood pressure of people suffering from atherosclerosis or hypertension. Diabetics on high dosages of insulin should only take vitamin E in graduated amounts.

As a precaution, anyone considering therapeutic doses of vitamin E should consult a nutritionist or a doctor trained in nutrition.

Of course, finding a doctor trained in nutrition can be a difficult problem. Most medical schools neglect nutritional subjects in their curricula. Those that teach nutrition usually offer it as an elective course only.

Although many doctors concerned with their health have studied nutrition on their own, the medical establishment generally considers vitamin therapy as too simplistic an approach to the treatment of diseases. Only recently have doctors from the Orthomolecular Society had success in publishing their findings in the established medical journals. They hope that as nutritional information becomes disseminated, acceptance of vitamin therapy will grow.

Meanwhile, the best supplementation plan for the older athlete is a complete range of vitamins and minerals, balanced according to individual needs.

Rate Your Protective Factors for Fitness

You can now see that several vitamins and minerals support your exercise program, increasing your endurance for the long run against aging.

Now turn to the building block for exercise, and see how you rate in this critical protective factor.

Building Block #4:

"Vitamin E and the Aging Jock:"
Your Protective Factors for Fitness

Occupation is primarily physical work (See p. 67) 34 points*	Exercises at least 1 hour daily 24 points*	Exercises at least 30 minutes daily 15 points*
Exercises at least 15 minutes daily 7 points*	Does not push self too hard 6 points	Eats vitamin E-rich foods (See p. 68) 5 points
Takes vitamin E daily (See p. 69) 4 points	Takes vitamin C daily (See p. 70) 3 points	Eats magnesium-rich foods (See p. 71) 2 points

Total the points for your present protective factors*

Your Score
Block #4 _____

---

*Score yourself for *only* the highest-value "exercise" square for which you qualify. The score for that square includes scores for all lower levels of exercise.

To page 94

for your next building block

5

SPEAKING OF CREAKING:

Arthritis: The Overlooked Role of Nutrition

Aches and Pains Provide Fertile Ground for Faddists

As we get older, our joints seem to have a tendency to get "rusty." According to the Arthritis Foundation, as many as 97 percent of persons over 60 have X-ray evidence of some arthritic changes, although not everyone experiences actual arthritic pain or other symptoms (Arthritis Foundation 1978). Arthritis is our nation's number one crippling disease, with more than *31.5 million* people in this country currently receiving treatment for it. The emotional costs of such widespread disability and pain are uncountable, but the dollar value of lost wages and medical bills connected with arthritic problems has been estimated at some *$13 billion a year!*

Obviously, with such vast sums of money at stake, and with arthritis's tremendous toll in human discomfort, it would not be surprising to see the modern-day equivalent of the old snake-oil peddlers rolling up in their circus wagons and hawking the latest thing in miracle cures. Indeed, many sufferers from arthritis have had their sufferings redoubled by exploitative quacks.

If we look at the facts it's easy to see why it is highly unlikely that there is a single panacea for all cases of arthritis. In its broadest sense, arthritis is simply defined as inflammation of a joint or joints. But this broad definition encompasses a great many quite different conditions, with different causes, clinical courses, and prognoses. It would be very surprising if there were one single cure for them all. Along with the established medical authorities, we should be suspicious of any "miracle cure" that claims to treat all arthritic conditions.

However, the established medical wisdom asserts that arthritis *cannot* be treated by *nutrition*, and that it is not in any way (with the exception of gout, one form of arthritis) a nutritionally related disease. On the contrary, we believe that arthritis, like most of the other diseases that strike with increasing frequency as our bodies begin to age, is very much connected with nutrition. But, since arthritis is a very complex group of diseases, the nutritional strategy for dealing with it can be equally complex.

A Large and Diverse Family of Diseases

Arthritis encompasses nearly a hundred different conditions, most of them chronic in nature. Three are by far the most common.

Osteoarthritis. The most widespread form is osteoarthritis, also known as degenerative joint disease—largely a result of the aging process; the accumulated wear and tear on the joints can result in pain and stiffness. But osteoarthritis is not usually a very disabling condition, and is generally not accompanied by the heat, swelling, or redness of inflammation. Osteoarthritis characteristically affects the weight-bearing joints—the knees and hips, for example—and may come on relatively early in life, affecting many women as they enter their forties. It often affects the fingers and toes as well, and has a greater tendency to develop in people who are overweight. While it's easy to see how the mechanical damage to weight-bearing joints would be greater in people who are carrying additional weight, it's not clear at present why the fingers and toes should also be affected. Bony protuberances, known as Heberden's nodes, may develop over the end joints of the fingers. The tendency to develop Heberden's nodes seems to run in families, as is the case with osteoarthritis in general.

Osteoarthritis is usually diagnosed on the basis of X-ray evidence, along with the patient's history and physical examination. Laboratory tests may help to rule out other forms of arthritis, since many blood tests are normal in osteoarthritis that are abnormal for other forms. There may be some changes in the synovial fluid in the joints, however.

As you might expect for a disease that results from structural damage to the joints, there is no cure for osteoarthritis. Pain relief is the objective in treatment, which may include drugs, heat, or corrective surgery. Sometimes in usual medical practice cortisone drugs are injected into the joints for temporary relief.

Rheumatoid arthritis. A much more puzzling disease is rheumatoid arthritis. There are many possible contributory factors. It appears to be partly hereditary, while at the same time connected with abnormal antibodies, perhaps related to some sort of viral or even protozoan involvement. Rheumatoid arthritis is characterized by inflammation, not only in the joints but also in the connective tissues throughout the body, so that it can affect the lungs, skin, blood vessels, muscles, spleen, and heart, and such joints as the hands and arms, hips, legs, and feet. Because of the generalized inflammatory nature of the disease, the rheumatoid arthritis sufferer may have fever, get tired easily, have a poor appetite, and be anemic; there may be enlargement of the lymph glands as well.

The disease often follows a peculiar pattern of flareups and remissions. The pain, stiffness, and swelling may go away for a while and then reappear, sometimes in a more severe form. Sometimes it may even disappear and never come back.

Rheumatoid arthritis tends to attack women more often than men, and affects children as well.

The disease is sometimes classified as one of the autoimmune diseases. In these diseases, generally associated with aging, the immune system begins to malfunction. Rather than attacking invading bacteria, it attacks the body's own cells and tissues. The autoimmune connection in rheumatoid arthritis is presently the subject of intensive investigation.

Diagnosing rheumatoid arthritis is nearly as tricky as explaining its cause. The so-called RA, or rheumatoid arthritis, factor, is found in the blood of a very high proportion of rheumatoid arthritis cases, but it is not definitely diagnostic of the disease, since there is a positive RA test in other diseases as well. Another blood test that may be done is the ANA, or antinuclear antibody test, as is the LE (lupus erythematosus) cell test. The synovial fluid from the affected joints may be examined, as may tissue samples from biopsies. X rays may also help to confirm the diagnosis.

The usual treatment of rheumatoid arthritis involves prescribing medication to reduce inflammation, a program of rest, special exercises, and physical therapy measures such as heat or splinting.

Gout. A third common form of arthritis is gouty arthritis, or simply gout. This condition apparently arises from an imbalance in the body's chemistry, often hereditary, and characterized by elevated levels of uric acid in the blood. Gout may also arise from the use of diuretic drugs. As a result of the metabolic defect, uric acid is produced in the body in greater quantities than the kidneys can excrete. The uric acid forms needlelike salt crystals that settle in the joints, leading to severe inflammation, often attacking the large joint of the big toe.

Certain foods, such as peas, beans, and liver, are high in their content of purines, which are substances that lead to the formation of uric acid in the body. When people affected by gout eat such foods, they have a tendency to develop elevated blood uric acid levels. In the past gout was often considered a disease of the privileged classes. This was probably partly true, since purine-rich foods tend to be those high in protein, such as meats and other dietary prerogatives of the affluent.

Gout may produce some changes that can be seen on X rays, but definitive diagnosis depends on the presence of elevated blood uric acid levels as well as an examination of the synovial fluid to determine the chemical composition of the crystals present in the joints. Another, similar condition known as pseudogout, also involves crystalline deposits in the joints, but in pseudogout the crystals are based on phosphates rather than on uric acid compounds.

Treatment of gout is directed at reducing the level of uric acid in the system, which is done through a combination of drugs such as colchicine, probenecid, and allopurinol, and control of the diet to reduce the intake of purines. Control of weight also seems to help keep uric acid levels down and prevent gout from flaring up.

Other forms of arthritis. Some of the other common arthritic conditions that affect adults are the following:

Ankylosing spondylitis is an inflammatory disease of the spine that is believed to be partly hereditary in nature; it may affect other joints as well.

Psoriatic arthritis is a form of arthritis associated with psoriasis.

Systemic lupus erythematosus, another "autoimmune disease," affects many of the body's tissues; in nine out of ten cases arthritis is one of the problems.

Bursitis is the inflammation of a bursa, or a fluid-containing sac that serves a cushioning function within a joint. Most commonly affected is the shoulder; also the hips and elbows.

Scleroderma is a disease of the connective tissue, characterized by thickening and hardening of the skin and by arthritic symptoms in the joints.

Infection can also produce arthritic symptoms, caused by bacterial invasion of the joints. Among the disease-causing organisms that can produce this type of arthritis are those that cause gonorrhea, meningitis, and tuberculosis. This type of arthritis will respond to appropriate antibiotic treatment.

Nutrition in the Treatment of Arthritis: The Ortho-dox View

Conventional medical authorities are unanimously con-servative concerning dietary approaches to arthritis. A leaflet distributed by the Arthritis Foundation is typical:

> The fact is, there is no valid scientific evidence that any dietary factor either causes or can help control arthritis. The only exceptions are in gout and when adjustments in a normal diet need to be made for an arthritis patient with an individual problem, such as overweight.
>
> (Arthritis Foundation)

We do not question the wisdom of warning against "miracle diets" which may promote a single food or a single nutrient at the expense of the varied mix of nutri-ents we all require. However, such statements may dis-courage arthritis sufferers from pursuing the very real possibility that in their own particular case their arthritis may be aggravated, complicated, or even caused, by a specific nutrient deficiency. Evidence is accumulating that different people's nutrient requirements are *not* the same, and that for many of us it may not be enough to simply stick religiously to the intake of the minimum daily re-quirements of the various nutrients.

Of course even the orthodox medical view empha-sizes good nutrition in the treatment of arthritis; but we believe that their definition of good nutrition may not go far enough. Before we look at some of the promising new nutritional approaches, let's review what the Arthritis Foun-dation and other medical authorities have to say.

Nutritionally related forms of arthritis. First of all, the conservative point of view recognizes that there *are* certain specific—though not very common—forms of ar-thritis that are related to nutritional factors. Vitamin C deficiency produces *scurvy,* one symptom of which may be bleeding into the joints, producing pain and swelling and thus arthriticlike symptoms. Restoration of vitamin C to the diet cures the problem. A rather exotic condition known as Kashin-Beck disease, produced by a toxic substance in a fungus that grows on grain, was noted in the nineteenth century in Siberia and northern China. A prominent symptom was swelling of the joints. Once the offending substance was identified and eliminated, the symptoms of the disease disappeared. A third form of arthritis that is somehow related to nutrition, is a swelling and pain in the joints which occurs in ten to twenty percent of patients who have undergone *intestinal bypass surgery* for obesity. Since the cause of this form of arthritis is unknown, the means of correcting it nutritionally is also unknown. It has been suggested that a change in intestinal bacteria may occur with the bypass surgery, resulting in the secretion of materials that cause the arthritis (Arthritis Foundation 1980).

Gout is routinely treated by diet. Of the three major forms of arthritis—rheumatoid, osteo-, and gouty—only gout is regularly treated partly by a dietary approach. While the therapy in gout relies heavily on drugs, diet is also important in reducing blood uric acid concentrations to normal, at least during acute flare-ups of the disease.

Owing to an inherited defect in the body's chemistry, it's necessary to readjust the diet of the gout sufferer to eliminate foods that are high in purine content. The current thinking is that dietary purines need no longer be restricted once serum uric acid concentrations have been returned to normal, which is brought about largely by the use of drugs.

Obesity can also contribute to high uric acid concentrations, and hence may bring on gout. Since many calorie-restricted reducing diets tend to emphasize foods high in protein, and hence high in purines, weight-reduction diets may need to be accompanied by increased doses of antigout drugs, and in any case should not be attempted during acute flare-ups of the condition. Overindulgence in alcohol can also trigger attacks in some gout patients.

The following is the Arthritis Foundation's "Low Purine Diet for Gout:"

Low Purine Diet for Gout

Avoid the Following:

1. Liver, sweetbreads, brains, kidney, anchovies, and sardines.
2. All meat extracts, gravies, and broths.
3. Asparagus, cauliflower, broccoli, mushrooms, dried beans (lima, kidney, and navy), lentils.
4. Chocolate, cocoa, and cola beverages.
5. Beer, ale, and red wine. Scotch whisky may usually be tolerated.
6. Whole grain cereals and oatmeals (any other cereal may be eaten). Use white bread or soybean bread.
7. Carbonated beverages.
8. Fresh peaches, apricots, and grapes.

You may notice that among the foods prohibited on the low-purine diet are some highly nutritious items such as liver, dried beans, whole grain cereals, oatmeal, sardines, and certain vitamin-rich fruits and vegetables. On the other hand, the recommended white bread is the nutritionist's classic nightmare. The gout patient is truly in a dilemma as to how to get an adequate diet while avoiding the high purine content of the prohibited foods.

Rheumatoid arthritis patients may not eat enough. In the treatment of rheumatoid and osteoarthritis the emphasis is on a well-balanced diet that provides an adequate supply of all nutrients. From the traditional medical point of view, this means daily intake from each of the four major food groups: (1) milk and dairy products; (2) meats; (3) vegetables and fruits; and (4) breads and cereals. Beyond this general prescription few specific recommendations are made. However, the nature of the disease may dictate special precautions in the diet of rheumatoid arthritis patients.

The RA patient, because he or she may feel sick all over, may have a poor appetite, and hence may not be getting an adequate supply of nutrients. Rheumatoid arthritis sufferers must therefore pay special attention to maintaining proper nutrition. The Arthritis Foundation

makes the following *limited case* for nutritional treatment
in rheumatoid arthritis:

> Thus, so far, no specific nutritional abnormality has
> been documented in rheumatoid arthritis. . . . Most
> doctors believe that careful attention should be paid to
> the nutritional status of any person with rheumatoid
> arthritis. For a number of reasons, people with rheuma-
> toid arthritis may be undernourished and develop defi-
> ciencies of metals, vitamins, amino acids or other
> nutrients. Restoration of the diet to normal frequently
> results in an improved sense of well being and better
> overall physical condition but cannot be expected to
> have any fundamental effect on the arthritic process
> itself.
>
> (Arthritis Foundation 1980)

Another problem for rheumatoid arthritis patients is
that they are commonly treated with large doses of
antiinflammatory drugs such as aspirin. Such drugs can
irritate the stomach, leading to peptic ulcer or gastritis,
which may be aggravated by fresh fruits and vegetables.
Dr. William Lages, in a leaflet distributed by the Arthritis
Foundation, recommends that canned or cooked fruits and
vegetables be used in this case, with supplementary vitamin C to replace the vitamin C lost in cooking. Alternatively,
antacids may be taken with meals, along with nonsteroidal
antiinflammatory drugs other than aspirin, with supplementary vitamins A, C, and D. Milk may soothe stomach
complaints for some patients; for those who must watch
their weight, Dr. Lages recommends low- or nonfat milk
products (Lages, no date).

We consider these recommendations to be a rather
artificial approach to diet, leading the patient away from
wholesome, natural foods toward a combination of chemicals.
It is hard to believe that a drug regimen, such as the
heavy use of aspirin or other painkillers, can be beneficial
to a patient if it turns nutritious food into an irritating
substance! Obviously, it would be desirable to find a better solution to the RA patient's dual needs of good nutrition and pain relief. We will explore some promising
nutritional leads in the last part of this chapter.

Weight control an objective in osteoarthritis. Obesity can contribute to, and seriously aggravate, the mechanical joint damage that leads to symptoms of osteoarthritis. To make matters worse, because. of pain and stiffness on movement, exercise and mobility may be limited, leading to even greater weight gain. The Arthritis Foundation therefore recommends careful monitoring of caloric intake for the osteoarthritis patient and weight reduction if indicated, concentrating on low-calorie foods such as lean meats, fish, vegetables, and fruits. We must remind anyone on a reducing diet, however, to be sure to supplement with vitamins and minerals that are not adequately provided in the reduced-calorie food allowances.

Arthritis: The Nutrition Connection

The medical establishment has largely abandoned any attempts to show a connection between arthritis and nutrition. In the heavily financed area of arthritis research, nutritional investigations receive very little attention. However, despite the pronouncements of orthodox medicine, nutritionists believe that dietary approaches may prove to be of paramount importance in the prevention and treatment of arthritis.

Arthritis associated with poor diet. Back in 1939, a dentist by the name of Dr. Weston Price carried out a monumental study entitled "Nutrition and Physical Degeneration; Isolated and Modernized Peoples," which disclosed a striking increase in bone and joint disease, as well as dental problems, as isolated cultures come into contact with Western civilization and begin to eat modern, "civilized" diets (Price 1970). As with so many modern "diseases of civilization," this study suggests that a first line of defense against arthritis is the restoration of important protective nutrients to our diet.

Dr. Robert Bingham, who advocates a nutritional approach to arthritis, reports that he has rarely seen a symptomatic case of arthritic disorders in patients with adequate dietary intakes. Hence, the proper treatment of these diseases must also include the correction of nutritional deficiencies and associated metabolic problems (Bingham 1972).

Dr. Roger Williams, a highly respected nutritionist, points out in *Nutrition Against Disease* (1981) that the synovial fluid that lubricates our joints is made up of mineral salts obtained from the diet, as well as mucoproteins that are manufactured by our cells from materials supplied in our food. It stands to reason, then, that if the proper building blocks are not supplied in the diet, the synovial fluid will not be able to perform its proper function of lubricating the joints.

Dr. Richard Kunin, in his book *Mega-Nutrition* (1980), sums up the position of the nutritionists succinctly when he says, "Don't believe anyone who tells you that arthritis is not a nutrition-related disease!"

A natural diet is essential. A good diet for the arthritis sufferer must begin with the components of a good diet for anyone—with the possible exception, of course, of the gout patient who may be unable to consume much protein and other purine-rich foods. We agree with the Arthritis Foundation that a varied, nutritious diet is desirable; but we would go further than the Arthritis Foundation and insist on *fresh, natural foods*, with the emphasis on raw or barely cooked vegetables and fresh fruits, plenty of protein and calcium (preferably from dairy products, which may be low-fat if weight control is desirable), and avoidance of all refined carbohydrates and excessive saturated fats.

Supplements may be vital to arthritics. While we should derive as much of our nutrient requirements as possible from natural foods, it is likely that many arthritis patients will benefit from additional nutrients in the form of vitamin and mineral supplementation.

One underlying factor in arthritis may be mineral imbalances. Mineral requirements vary considerably from one individual to another. One way to detect possible mineral deficiencies is through an analysis of your blood. Laboratory investigation of the synovial fluid may also reveal mineral imbalances that can be corrected through diet and supplementation.

Calcium deposits form in joints that are subjected to wear and tear or are inflamed. These calcium deposits eventually distort the joints and lead to the characteristic pain and stiffness of arthritis. Some of the calcium that collects in these deposits in the joints is actually "stolen" from adjacent bone. This is one good reason why arthritis patients should be sure to maintain an adequate calcium intake. Even if not enough calcium is supplied in the diet (preferably in the form of milk and other dairy products, as well as perhaps the cooking and gnawing of bones and other animal sources of calcium), calcium deposits will still form in the joints, at the expense of the composition of the bones. So the bones are weakened at the same time that the joints are damaged.

Other excellent sources of calcium besides milk are hard cheeses, soft fish bones (salmon, sardines, and herring), and dark green leafy vegetables; other, slightly less rich sources of calcium include softer cheeses, dried figs, dried legumes, baked beans, and broccoli.

Some people tend to overdose themselves with calcium supplements unbalanced with magnesium. This leads to a condition known as hypercalcemia, or elevated blood calcium, which in turn leads to the formation of calcium deposits in the joints. Magnesium is more chemically active than calcium, and magnesium salts may help to prevent or reverse the buildup of calcium-salt deposits in the joints. Recent research has shown that magnesium-based intradermal salves, when applied to the skin, have been successful in dissolving calcium deposits in the underlying joints.

Magnesium occurs naturally in a variety of foods including shellfish, nuts, seeds, and green leafy vegetables. A good calcium-magnesium supplement such as dolomite may also prove helpful. Magnesium also protects against the development of atherosclerotic deposits in the aorta, a condition that often accompanies arthritis; and so, as in the case of most crucial nutrients, this mineral serves a variety of protective purposes.

Another mineral that appears to play a prominent role in arthritic disorders is *copper*. A higher than normal copper content has been noted in the blood and joint fluid of patients with rheumatoid arthritis. Cortisone, which is often prescribed for relief of arthritic symptoms, may also bring about a lowering of these elevated copper levels. Certain amino acids such as penicillamine and histidine, bind to copper in the body, removing it through the urine. These have also provided relief in some cases of arthritis. However, some zinc is also removed by these amino acids, and so zinc may need to be supplemented when they are used.

Many arthritis sufferers report that they obtain relief from wearing copper bracelets; it is possible that the metal may be absorbed directly through the skin, somehow influencing a disturbed copper metabolism. While we certainly cannot guarantee that any of these approaches will work for everyone, they do point to the importance of copper in at least some cases of arthritis.

Zinc levels tend to be very low in rheumatoid arthritis patients. This is another mineral element that appears to help repair inflamed and damaged arthritic tissues in some people. Patients receiving cuprimine (penicillamine) or other chelating agents, should be sure they are maintaining adequate zinc levels. A sign of zinc deficiency is a loss of the sense of taste.

Selenium, one of the valuable "antiaging" substances, useful for its antioxidant and free-radical-deactivating properties, has also been shown to have a therapeutic effect in rheumatoid and osteoarthritis, perhaps through its enhancement of immune functioning (Weiner 1981, p. 90). If adequate selenium cannot be obtained in the diet through selenium-rich foods such as brewer's yeast, mushrooms, asparagus, garlic, and whole grains, then a careful dosage regimen can be worked out under medical supervision. Remember that selenium is highly toxic when taken in excess.

Osteoporosis: a threat to aging bones. A very common problem of mineral utilization among older people is osteoporosis, or loss of calcium from the bones. This condition makes the bones so brittle and fragile that they may fracture very easily, and hence protecting the calcium content of your bones can be a truly life-saving objective. Because osteoporosis is particularly prevalent among older women, we will be discussing the dietary prevention of this condition in chapter 6, which addresses the special problems of aging that confront women—but obviously, there is a message there for men as well!

Vitamin supplements help some arthritis sufferers. As with minerals, individuals vary greatly in their need for various vitamins, sometimes far exceeding the Recommended Dietary Allowances; there is evidence that in some arthritis patients massive doses of certain vitamins may have a beneficial effect.

Dr. William Kaufman found that megadoses of *niacinamide* greatly improved joint flexibility in a large group of patients he studied (Kaufman 1949). He prescribed this B vitamin in large doses, ranging from 400 to 2,250 milligrams a day. Another form, *niacin*, has also been used. Dr. Richard Kunin recommends giving niacin at the dosage level where it just begins to produce the characteristic side effect of flushing. Niacinamide is preferred by many patients because it does *not* produce this flushing response.

Vitamin C is another of the extremely versatile "antiaging" vitamins. Some cases of arthritis, as well as back pain, have reportedly been greatly relieved by large doses of vitamin C. Besides its general protective effects as an antioxidant and free radical scavenger, vitamin C promotes the production of collagen, the connective-tissue material that the body needs to repair damaged joints. Dr. Carl Pfeiffer (1975) says that arthritics may benefit from a combination of 100 milligrams of niacin and 500 milligrams of vitamin C, with meals, taken three times a day. The niacin dose is lower than that used by Dr. Kaufman, but is better tolerated (Pfeiffer 1975, p. 453).

Pantothenic acid, another of the B vitamins, was found in an English study to be deficient in the blood of some rheumatoid arthritis patients, in direct proportion to the severity of their arthritic complaints (Barton-Wright and Elliott 1963). Treatment of these patients with pantothenic acid brought short-term relief, indicating that this B vitamin may be helpful in arthritis but that it isn't the final answer.

Vitamin B_6 was found by Dr. John Ellis to relieve arthritic symptoms, particularly pain, stiffness, and locking of the finger joints. Other studies have suggested that vitamin B_6 may help to remedy an error in tryptophan metabolism that is found in many arthritis patients (Williams 1981, p. 132).

The B vitamin *riboflavin* has also been recommended as a supplement for arthritis sufferers, as has *vitamin A*.

Avoiding the dangers of aspirin and cortisone. Besides these minerals and vitamins, a number of other dietary adjuncts have been found to be helpful in some cases of arthritis. An important element of the conventional treatment of arthritis is the use of pain-killing medications and antiinflammatory drugs—most commonly aspirin, and in more severe cases, cortisone. Such medications can have a negative effect on nutrition and overall health. Aspirin is well-known for its ability to produce gastritis, which may discourage proper food intake or make the arthritis sufferer intolerant to many nutritious foods. Cortisone has many seriously damaging effects when used on a long-term, chronic basis, and may actually depress endocrine activity to the point where the body is no longer able to manufacture its own cortisone. If at all possible, it is advisable to avoid cortisone altogether and to replace aspirin with more natural means of pain relief.

Kunin (1980) reports that many patients obtain relief with *copper aspirinate*, a form of aspirin combined with copper, which reportedly has much greater cortisonelike activity than aspirin alone, while the copper helps to protect against the irritating effects of aspirin on the stomach. Dr. Kunin also reports that many patients benefit from the amino acid *tryptophan*, available in health food stores, as a means of pain relief and tranquilization.

A food supplement now available in tablet form that shows cortisonelike antiinflammatory activity is *yucca plant saponin*. American Indians have been using the yucca plant for centuries as a foodstuff, which testifies to its safety. Yucca saponin has been given in tablet extract form as a dietary supplement to arthritis patients, with reported relief of pain, swelling, and stiffness. An incidental finding in one study by Bingham and co-workers was a reduction of blood cholesterol level in some of the patients given yucca saponin. Obviously this natural antiinflammatory and pain reliever warrants further investigation. Yucca saponin apparently produces its beneficial effects through its influence on the intestinal bacteria (Bingham et al.).

Rate Your Protective Factors Against Arthritis

As you can see, diet and nutrient supplements *can* reverse *some* arthritic conditions. More importantly, if you will eat the right foods and take your insurance allotment of vitamins and minerals, you can probably avoid becoming one of those millions of older people who suffer from this joint disease. Look in the building block for your keys to avoiding painful, swollen joints.

Building Block #5:

"Speaking of Creaking:"
Your Protective Factors Against Arthritis

Keeps weight within 10% of ideal (See p. 84) 10 points	Fruits & vegetables make up 50% of the diet (See p. 88) 9 points	Avoids excess animal fats (See p. 88) 8 points
Gets adequate calcium foods (See p. 88) 7 points	Gets adequate magnesium foods (See p. 89) 6 points	Takes vitamin C supplement (See p. 83) 5 points
Takes pantothenic acid supplement (See p. 91) 4 points	Takes niacin supplement (See p. 91) 3 points	Takes vitamin B_6 supplement (See p. 91) 2 points

Total the points for your present protective factors.

Your Score Block #5 _____

To page 112 (women) *or* 118 (men)

for your next building block

6

GIRLS NO MORE:

For Women Only

Menopause: A Uniquely Human Stage of Life?

Of all the mammals on earth, the human female has long been thought the only one who stops ovulating and menstruating in midlife. Recent observations of langurs and macaques suggest that perhaps these primates, too, lose their fertility late in life. But certainly its emotional overtones make the human menopause a unique experience.

There is probably an evolutionary reason for the human menopause. Perhaps it's to guarantee that her offspring will not be left without protection and support during their long period of dependency; thus, a woman loses the ability to produce still more babies well before the end of her life.

Generally occurring sometime between the ages of forty and fifty-five, menopause consists of a gradual cessation of menstruation, with periods becoming increasingly irregular and less frequent. Accompanying the termination of the monthly cycles is a decreased production of the female hormones estrogen and progesterone. Because of the changes in hormone levels women may experience a variety of sometimes unpleasant symptoms. There is undoubtedly a psychological element as well in many women's symptomatology; for what more irrevocable reminder could there be that one is growing older, than to lose the ability to reproduce?

It is conceivable that if we learn how to extend the human life span, women in the future may be able to bear children later in life. This would be particularly welcome among those who are now postponing their families until well into their thirties, or even beyond. Although we cannot presently suggest any way to reverse menopause itself, we can suggest some strategies for reducing some of the symptoms and hazards of this important transitional period in a woman's life.

Symptoms and Diseases of Menopause

Actually, only about twenty-five percent of American women experience significant symptoms during menopause, other than the cessation of ovulation and menstruation. Among the unpleasant symptoms reported by this minority are those related to vasomotor instability, including hot flushes and sweats, especially night sweats. Other symptoms are psychological in nature, such as depression, irritability, crying spells, insomnia, and fatigue. Dryness of the vagina and a resultant discomfort on intercourse are other common complaints.

The diseases of midlife strike particularly hard at women. Up until this time, for example, women have a much lower incidence of heart disease than do their male counterparts. But now, during menopause, women become more susceptible to many chronic degenerative diseases, including diabetes, high blood pressure, ischemic heart disease, and osteoporosis. Some of these diseases become more prominent partly because of the reduced production of estrogen. The hormone actually protects premenopausal women against calcium loss, and probably some aspects of heart disease.

The estrogen controversy. Because estrogen protects against osteoporosis and other chronic degenerative diseases, many doctors prescribe this female hormone to their middle-aged female patients. Dr. Carlton Fredericks in his excellent book, *Breast Cancer: A Nutritional Approach* (1977) traces the history of this hormone's use in modern medicine. Estrogen replacement therapy became popular during the 1960s, and now it represents some fifty million dollars a year in prescriptions, with an estimated three million American women taking Premarin, the most widely prescribed estrogen replacement. In addition to the protection it affords against the diseases of midlife, estrogen replacement therapy often produces "miraculous" reversals of such menopausal complaints as vaginal dryness and flushes.

Unfortunately, there's a catch. It has now been shown beyond any doubt that estrogen replacement therapy greatly increases the chances of cancer of the breast and uterus. Even those doctors who advocate estrogen therapy now say that it should be used sparingly, and only for short periods of time, and that women on estrogen should be followed with annual Pap smears and breast exams, and uterine biopsies where indicated.

Women often justly complain that the medical establishment, being largely dominated by males, does not always have the best interests of female patients in mind when treating disorders unique to the female sex. Certainly the use of estrogen therapy seems to fit this criticism. Listen to what some of our physicians are saying to justify the serious risks of estrogen treatment as a means of preventing osteoporosis:

> The cancer produced by estrogen is curable. Osteoporosis is not. It's a trade-off.

> What we are talking about is saving women a lot of pain and deformity and fracture.
>   (Both quotes from *Time* 1981)

We would hardly agree that cancer is "curable." The current "cure" for breast cancer is still mutilating surgery, usually followed by radiation therapy and chemotherapy that have many devastating side effects. Is exchanging the pain and deformity of cancer a fair trade for the pain, deformity, and fracture of osteoporosis? Certainly there must be a better solution!

Nutritional Approaches to the Problems of Menopause

Fortunately, there *is* a gentler, safer approach, and one that promotes health and long life for the whole woman, rather than merely loading her with drugs and assuring her that any resultant cancerous growth can be handily lopped off. For the symptoms of menopause, there is in fact no better solution than a sound program of nutrition, accompanied by adequate exercise and relaxation.

Let's look first at nutritional strategies for treating some of the specific symptoms of menopause, and then we'll outline broad recommendations for optimal diet and supplementation during this delicate transitional period in a woman's life. These nutritional treatments will not only alleviate specific menopausal problems, but they will also promote overall good health, protect against chronic degenerative diseases that come on with aging, and hopefully, slow down the aging process itself.

Hot flushes and sweats. "Hot flashes," of all the disturbances of menopause, are those most familiar to the general public—and most often joked about by younger people and men of all ages. Such symptoms are caused by a disturbance of the vasomotor nerves, as Gail Sheehy clearly explains in her treatment of menopause in *Passages:*

> What is happening when waves of heat spread over the upper body, often followed by chills? The medical term is *vasomotor instability*. The vasomotor nerves are responsible for enlarging or decreasing the diameter of the blood vessels. Ordinarily, these nerves will take their cue from the body temperature. . . . But when hormones become unstable, they disturb the signals going to the vasomotor nerves. Dizziness, too, in the middle-aged woman or man, is usually caused by some disturbance of blood flow caused by the agi-

tated vasomotor nerves. The palpitating heart can have the same cause.

(Sheehy 1977, p. 463)

The annoying flushing and sweating will eventually subside as your body becomes accustomed to lower levels of hormones. In the meantime, vitamin E at a dosage level from 400 to 1,600 international units (IU) daily has been shown to help in many cases. (One caution concerning vitamin E: Some people with high blood pressure experience a rise in pressure when they take supplemental vitamin E. If you have high blood pressure, increase your vitamin E intake cautiously, under your doctor's supervision.) In addition to this invaluable vitamin, regular exercise, adequate sleep, and regular relaxation such as yoga or meditation, have been shown to alleviate the severity of flushing.

Flushes and sweats can be aggravated by caffeine and alcohol, so cutting down or eliminating these beverages may help. We will recommend some herbal substitutes later on, in our discussion of diet. Also, smoking causes the ovaries to produce fewer hormones, and may even induce early menopause and more severe symptoms. This is a very good reason to quit smoking at this time of life, if you haven't already done so. While we certainly wouldn't advocate being overweight, it may help to bring your weight up to normal if you're overly thin, since some natural estrogens are produced by the body's fat stores, and may help to maintain your hormonal balance.

Depression and irritability. The psychological symptoms of menopause can be very real and distressing. Vitamin E has been found useful in helping to alleviate these problems. In addition, giving up caffeine will help relieve irritability—and this means not only coffee and tea, but also cola drinks and other caffeine-containing soft drinks!

Vaginal dryness and soreness. Reduced estrogen levels may cause the mucous membranes of the vagina to become dry, resulting in discomfort during intercourse for some women. All the recommendations for eliminating hot flushes—taking vitamin E, adjusting your diet, quitting smoking, and avoiding being underweight, can be of help for this problem. There are many oils, creams, and lotions that can be used to enhance lubrication. Try using an unscented lubricating cream, A&D ointment, baby oil, vitamin E oil, or pure aloe gel. There are estrogen-containing creams available, but we recommend *against* these for the same reasons we would discourage the use of oral estrogen therapy.

This may be an opportunity for you and your partner to explore some alternatives to vaginal intercourse that can be equally stimulating and satisfying expressions of your love. Remember this: Surveys have shown that older women who have continued to engage regularly in sexual activity throughout their lives are much less likely to develop vaginal dryness—a good argument for keeping in shape sexually as well as physically (Starr and Weiner 1981)!

Preventing Osteoporosis

One of the most unspectacular processes that begins in women with menopause is osteoporosis. In terms of its crippling and life-threatening potential, however, this condition is one of the most serious threats to older women, and one that they must take specific precautions to prevent.

How estrogen influences bone loss. With decreasing production of estrogen, women are at an increased risk of developing osteoporosis, or thinning of the bones due to loss of calcium. Normally, as old bones are broken down, or resorbed, new bone tissue is manufactured to compensate for the loss. Estrogen helps regulate this production of new bones, and if it is deficient, the rate of bone replacement is not fast enough to keep up with resorption. Porous, brittle bones can lead to the collapse of vertebrae with a resultant loss of height, and back pain, as well as susceptibility to fractures. Some 200,000 older Americans— most of them women—suffer fractured hips each year. Many become permanently disabled by hip fractures, and many die from complications following such injuries or surgical treatment.

Calcium-rich diet a must. It is extremely important, therefore, for women approaching midlife to ensure that they are receiving an adequate supply of calcium. The diet should supply plenty of calcium-rich foods, including milk, yogurt, and cheese; choose nonfat and low-fat dairy products if you are watching your weight or otherwise limiting your fat intake. Other good sources of calcium include sunflower and sesame seeds (these, however, are also high in fat!), corn tortillas, soybean and tofu, kale, broccoli, and mustard and collard greens. Women after menopause require even more calcium than young people require at puberty, when the bones are undergoing rapid growth. To ensure adequate calcium intake it will generally be necessary for some women to supplement dietary calcium with approximately 1,000 milligrams of calcium a day, plus 400 IU of vitamin D to promote calcium absorption.

High-protein diet induces calcium loss. It has been shown that high protein consumption actually *increases* the loss of calcium from the bones. For this reason, women approaching midlife should limit their intake of meat, poultry, and fish. Not only will this reduce your protein intake, but it will also decrease your consumption of the fat that accompanies protein in animal sources. Add more vegetable sources—a complementary combination of beans, whole grains, and other vegetables—as well as dairy products and eggs for your main supply of protein.

Exercise helps prevent osteoporosis. Studies have also shown that exercise is essential in preventing osteoporosis. Research initiated by the American space program to determine the effects of immobility and weightlessness on our astronauts demonstrated that lack of activity causes the calcium to pour out of the bones. Higher-than-average skeletal density has been observed in cross-country runners and ballet dancers, and in the dominant hand as compared to the nondominant one. The explanation seems to lie in the level of activity (Sandler and Herbert 1981). One of the best safeguards against calcium loss is thus a regular exercise program.

In addition, tobacco smoking and excessive alcohol consumption have been associated with increased osteoporosis, and heavy coffee drinking is also suspect—so change your habits and protect your bones from this dangerous and debilitating condition!

New hope from fluoride treatment. As we have already observed, many doctors are unfortunately overly eager to prescribe estrogen as a means of slowing down the loss of calcium from the bones. If you follow the dietary and life-style recommendations we have given, you should not need to resort to this potentially dangerous form of treatment. A promising approach currently under study is the use of large doses of sodium fluoride combined with calcium to stimulate the production of new bone. The fluoride seems to be as effective as estrogen in maintaining a favorable balance between bone growth and resorption. Fluoride and calcium treatment may prove to be a helpful preventative measure in the future.

Protecting Against Breast and Uterine Cancer and Related Problems

Breast cancer is probably the disease of midlife most dreaded by women. Although more and more women appear to be surviving, largely owing to earlier detection, the conventional treatment of choice in breast cancer remains a combination of mutilating surgery and dangerous drug and radiation therapy. Given the limited options available once the disease has developed, prevention—if it is possible—is a paramount concern.

Correct diet protects against estrogen effects. While there does appear to be a hereditary element, it takes more than just heredity to produce a case of breast or endometrial cancer. One factor that seems to play an important role is diet. Japanese women, for example, have only about twenty percent the rate of breast cancer that American women do. When these Oriental women move to Hawaii, however, and eat the "American" diet for about ten years, their incidence of cancer becomes the same as for American women (Fredericks 1977).

Does the change in diet result in the loss of a protective factor against cancer? Nutritionist Carlton Fredericks, among others, thinks this is the case. In *Breast Cancer: A Nutritional Approach,* he points to evidence that indicates that dietary factors protect against the dangers of estrogen.

About one third of all breast cancers are stimulated by the presence of excess estrogen. This is a very good reason to refuse estrogen replacement therapy for menopausal symptoms, just as younger women should avoid the added risk of cancer from contraceptive pills containing estrogen. After menopause, many women think it is safe to take estrogen because their bodies are no longer producing the hormone at the same rate as younger women's bodies. This reasoning is incorrect. Many studies have shown that estrogen medication increases the risk of developing breast and uterine cancer regardless of the woman's hormone production.

Even if women avoid the added risk of estrogen therapy, however, there are other sources of estrogen that are relatively unavoidable, including that produced by the supporting tissues of the ovaries and by the body's stores of fat. Certain foods are also sources of estrogen, including whole grains and meat from animals that have been deliberately *fed* estrogen—most notably beef.

B complex vitamins help the liver detoxify estrogen. Since estrogen intake, in some form or other, is virtually unavoidable, it is important for women to follow a diet that will protect against its dangers. One way that diet can help to protect against cancer is by promoting the liver's activity in converting the potentially harmful estrogen into a harmless substance known as estriol. Vitamin B complex is particularly important in keeping the liver well nourished so that it can carry out the important work of deactivating estrogen in the body. Women whose diets have been chronically deficient in vitamin B complex may have greatly increased vitamin B requirements for the rest of their lives.

Not all the B complex vitamins have been identified at this point, and so it is important to eat foods that are rich in B vitamins (such as wheat germ and organ meats), since unknown factors can't be put into supplemental tablets. The following is a list of the currently known constituents of the B complex:

Thiamin (B_1)   Inositol
Riboflavin (B_2)   Choline

Biotin   Pangamic acid (B_{15})
Niacin, niacinamide (B_3)   Hydroxycobalamin,
Pyridoxine (B_6)   cyanocobalamin (B_{12})
Para-aminobenzoic acid   Orotic acid (B_{13})
   (PABA)
Folic acid

(Fredericks 1977, p. 62)

Of the B vitamins, the most important for supporting the liver's conversion of estrogen into estriol are *inositol* and *choline*. Unfortunately, most B complex supplements don't contain adequate amounts of these important vitamins, and so additional supplementation may be required. You can buy these B vitamins separately at a health food store or pharmacy. A daily intake of 500 milligrams of inositol and 1,000 milligrams of choline is recommended by Carlton Fredericks.

Lecithin is another important nutrient among whose many functions is the control of cholesterol, so that it helps to prevent atherosclerotic deposits in the arteries. Lecithin also seems to help support the liver's control of estrogen activity. Naturally occurring in polyunsaturated fats, lecithin may be supplied adequately if your diet is rich in milk, eggs, soybeans, and whole grains. Unfortunately, like so many protective nutrients, lecithin is generally removed in the processing of vegetable oils. For this reason, cold-pressed oils are preferred. Lecithin may be taken as a supplement in the form of granules which can be mixed into your cereal or juice. It is also available in capsules. If you take lecithin, you can reduce your inositol and choline supplementation somewhat since these B vitamins are contained in lecithin.

Other nutrients. Thyroid function is also related to estrogen production. When thyroid hormone levels are low, estrogen levels are likely to be high. Adequate intake of iodine is therefore essential to promote proper activity of the thyroid. A correct diet to help estrogen control, as well as vitamin B_1 (thiamine) and about 100 micrograms of iodine daily (supplied in such sources as kelp tablets), will ensure normal functioning of a healthy thyroid gland.

As we saw in chapter 2, antioxidants are also important in protecting against cancer. Vitamin E, vitamin C, and selenium, along with vitamin A, all have significant anticancer properties. Vitamin E has also been shown to relieve soreness and to reduce nodule size in cystic breast disease, which is usually benign but may be a precancerous condition. In younger women, this estrogen-controlling program has also been shown to alleviate premenstrual symptoms, both physical and psychological.

Some cautions concerning antiestrogen diets. For younger women who adopt the antiestrogen diet to control premenstrual symptoms, remember that it may take several months for the symptoms to abate. Dr. Fredericks explains that because adequate diet may first stimulate hormonal functioning, there may be an initial *increase* in estrogen production, producing an *aggravation* of the symptoms. Later, as the liver is stimulated to function properly in converting this estrogen into estriol, the estrogen-related symptomatology will abate.

One further warning is in order. These dietary recommendations are for women who are presently *healthy*. If you have cystic disease or any other precancerous or cancerous condition, don't run the risk of treating yourself. Even if you are healthy, seek guidance from a doctor who understands the importance of nutrition and will help you to devise a nutritional program adapted to your special needs.

General Dietary Recommendations for Menopause

The body undergoes profound changes during menopause. It should come as no surprise, then, that your diet should be adjusted to reflect your new nutritional needs. The following recommendations will help you to design your dietary plan at midlife.

Avoid being overweight. Be careful to watch your weight during and after menopause. With decreasing estrogen production, the risk of heart disease increases greatly, and one of the most serious risk factors in heart disease is obesity. Remember also that if you're on a reducing diet you are getting fewer of the vitamins and minerals your body needs. Vitamin and mineral supplements become even more important if you're cutting back on your calories.

Eat fresh, natural foods, emphasizing plant sources. To ensure that you get as many protective vitamins and minerals as possible from your foods, eat plenty of fresh fruits and vegetables, including whole grains and legumes as complementary protein sources. Such a diet also assures high-fiber intake, which will protect against constipation and many chronic diseases, as we will see in chapter 8. Avoid refined carbohydrates (white flour and white sugar), and canned fruits and vegetables. Eat vegetables raw or lightly steamed, never overly cooked, and retain the skins whenever possible. Be sure to include root vegetables in your diet, including potatoes, baked or boiled with the skins on.

Reduce your protein intake. Because high protein intake contributes to calcium loss from the bones, you should reduce your consumption of meat, fish, and poultry. To avoid the fat that accompanies these foods, never eat poultry skins, and trim all visible fat from meat before cooking. Avoid processed and smoked meats such as bacon, ham, luncheon meats, and all other products containing nitrates and nitrites, which can lead to the formation of cancer-causing nitrosamines in the body. Your protein can be adequately supplied by complementary vegetable sources such as whole grains and beans, and if you consume eggs and dairy products as well, you will get all the essential amino acids even without using complementary protein sources.

Don't be afraid to use dairy products. For calorie control, emphasize low-fat or nonfat dairy products such as yogurt, low-fat milk, and hard cheeses made from skim milk. These will supply calcium, so important in preventing osteoporosis, as well as protein and valuable vitamins. Avoid dairy products high in fat, such as cream, sour cream, ice cream, butter, and whole-milk hard cheeses. Cottage cheese may be low in calories, but it's also low in calcium owing to processing.

Be wary of fats. After menopause women are at a greatly increased risk of developing atherosclerosis and heart disease. While it has not been conclusively demon-

strated that cholesterol in the diet raises blood cholesterol
levels and increases the risk of cardiovascular disease, we
recommend that you be cautious in your intake of saturated fats. Of course, fats also contribute to obesity. Remember also, that overemphasizing polyunsaturated fats
in the diet can contribute to the risk of developing cancer,
so moderation must be practiced in all your fat intake.

As for eggs, the cholesterol scare has caused many
people to avoid this nutritious "superfood." While it is
probably wise to restrict your intake of eggs to reasonable
limits, we certainly wouldn't discourage their use entirely,
since they are such a rich source of valuable nutrients.
Cooking methods may influence the relative potential dangers of eggs. For a complete discussion of this subject, see
"Eggs, angiotoxins, and heart attacks" beginning on page
28 in chapter 1.

If you have elevated lipoproteins in your blood, follow
your doctor's advice. You may need to severely limit or
entirely eliminate your intake of eggs.

Avoid refined sugar. At this time in your life, when
all the food you consume must really count toward your
overall nutrition, there is no excuse for consuming the
"empty calories" of refined sugar. Besides contributing to
obesity and discouraging the intake of more nutritious
foods, sugar actually depletes B vitamins in the body,
since it requires these vitamins in order to be burned.
Sugar in the diet also has the effect of raising blood lipid
levels in women after menopause, thereby increasing the
risk of atherosclerosis and heart disease.

If you have a craving for sweets, try eating fruit
instead. These natural foods will also provide the additional benefits of fiber. According to Dr. Carlton Fredericks,
a craving for sugar can sometimes be overcome by high
doses of vitamins B_6 and C (as much as a gram of each per
day). Dr. Fredericks believes that sugar cravings are really
a sign of an unrecognized allergy (Fredericks 1977, pp.
96–97).

Remember that processed foods contain large quantities of "hidden sugars"—another reason to emphasize fresh
foods. If you *must* sometimes use processed foods, learn to

read the labels carefully to identify the sugars that are listed under many guises.

Restrict salt intake. Table salt, or sodium chloride, really doesn't belong on your table at this time in your life. Natural foods contain plenty of sodium to meet your body's needs. Sodium increases blood pressure, which can lead to a host of other deadly problems. In order to maintain the balance between sodium and potassium your body requires, eat fruits and vegetables to increase your potassium intake. Avoid processed foods, which generally contain much too much salt.

It may seem difficult to eliminate salt from your cooking. The desire for salt is actually an acquired taste; your taste buds develop a tolerance for the salty flavor, and so you are tempted to add ever-increasing quantities to your food. Try substituting herbs, lemon juice, and other flavors rather than depending on this unnecessary condiment.

Use alcohol moderately or not at all. A glass of wine can be a fine complement to your diet if you can keep your consumption to a very moderate level. Alcohol in any amount, however, may aggravate the flushing of menopause, in which case it should be avoided. Remember that alcohol contains calories, and so excessive alcohol consumption can contribute to obesity. If you have a problem limiting your drinking, don't drink alcohol at all; and in any case, hard liquor must be avoided.

Break your caffeine habit. Coffee, tea, cola drinks, and chocolate all contain caffeine. Not only does caffeine often aggravate the symptoms of flushing and sweats, but it can make menopause even harder on your nerves.

There are many excellent herbal or cereal-based teas that you can drink instead of caffeine-containing products. An herbal tea that is particularly helpful for the symptoms of menopause, such as flushing and sweating, consists of a blend of one part each of chamomile, peppermint, and red clover tops. Steep five minutes and drink warm. For irritability and nervousness that may accompany menopause, a soothing herbal tea may be made from passionflower, chamomile, scullcap, hibiscus, or valerian, flavored with sassafras or sarsaparilla root.

Breaking the caffeine habit can be a trying experience, as can changing any other lifelong pattern such as alcohol use or smoking. To make it as easy on yourself as possible, we recommend that you begin immediately to improve your nutritional status by following our suggestions for diet and supplementation, so that you will be in the strongest, most resilient condition as you wean yourself away from your dependencies.

Special Supplements for Women

Women during menopause generally require vitamin and mineral supplementation to ensure adequate supplies of essential nutrients. Table 6.1 summarizes the specific recommendations we have made in this chapter for a

Table 6.1

Vitamin/Mineral Supplementation for Menopause

Supplement	Function
Vitamin E	Protects against hot flushes & psychological symptoms; may relieve vaginal dryness; protects against breast lumps & cancer
Vitamin C	Must be taken with vitamin E for best effect
Vitamin B complex: Inositol Choline	Support liver function to deactivate estrogen & protect against cancer
B_1 (thiamine)	Supports thyroid function
Iodine	Supports thyroid function
Calcium	Promotes new bone growth to offset calcium loss from bones
Vitamin D	Promotes calcium absorption

carefully planned diet for midlife and beyond. Of course the protective nutrients listed have other important functions as well as those related to menopausal problems. You may require other supplements as well to promote good health and protect against the diseases of aging.

For overall protection, one approach is to take a multivitamin/mineral supplement daily. The best strategy is to find one that supplies approximately the minimum daily requirement of all essential vitamins and minerals, and then to take *additional* amounts of these important nutrients, if they are not adequately supplied in the single supplement pill.

The most important thing to bear in mind concerning supplementation is that it is just that—an *addition* to your daily diet, not a substitute for wise eating. Your first and most important source of vitamins and minerals should be your food—particularly since we have not yet identified all the essential nutrients, and so these unknown factors cannot be supplied in the form of a pill.

Remember also, that "superfoods" such as wheat germ, brewer's yeast, organ meats, eggs, and dairy products, contain concentrated quantities of important vitamins and minerals, and should be incorporated into your diet.

Smoking Contributes to Problems of Aging

If you are still a smoker as you enter midlife, this is an important time to quit this dangerous habit. Not only does smoking contribute to the risk of cancer, heart disease, and emphysema, but it increases the risk of osteoporosis and may produce menopause at an earlier date. If that isn't reason enough to give up smoking, remember that smokers have more wrinkles than nonsmokers!

The Importance of Exercise

A sound nutrition program for menopause must be accompanied by a carefully planned and conscientiously carried out program of exercise, done every day, for maximum benefits. If you are not normally active, such an exercise program should include strenuous, aerobic activities such as jogging, bicycling, hiking, dancing, or swimming; stretching and flexibility exercises; and strengthening exercises in which you exert effort against resistance, such as certain calisthenics or weight training. Of course, if your normal activities include daily physical exertion, your need for a "formal" exercise program is diminished correspondingly.

Besides helping to keep your weight under control, regular exercise will help to alleviate many of the symptoms of menopause such as flushes and mental irritability, and is essential for the prevention of osteoporosis.

Rate Your Protective Factors for Menopause

Menopause need not be that dark corner of life that so many women have come to fear. By following a few reasonable dietary strategies and taking a few supplements, life can begin anew. Now let's look at your building block to see how well you are protecting yourself against the special problems of menopause.

Building Block #6:

"Girls No More:"
Your Protective Factors for Menopause

Does not take estrogen (See p. 96) 10 points	Takes calcium (See p. 100) 9 points	Eats natural, high-fiber foods—at least 50% of diet (See p. 106) 8 points
Limits fats & meats in diet (See pp. 106–107) 7 points	Does not smoke (See p. 101) 6 points	Takes vitamins E & C (See p. 99) 5 points
Exercises regularly (See p. 101) 4 points	Takes vitamin B complex, inositol, & choline (See p. 103) 3 points	Handles stress without tranquilizers (See p. 99) 2 points

Total the points for your present   Your Score
protective factors.   Block #6 _____

To page 118

for your next building block

7

(NOT) FOR MEN ONLY:

Potency, Virility, and the Prostate

One of the most difficult subjects to discuss from a medical viewpoint with any certainty is male potency—or the absence of it! Men are not overly enthusiastic about admitting their troubles in this department.

Nevertheless, there *are* certain knowns. And these methods for restoring potency, virility, and other sexual deficits, are available to you simply, and *without* costly prescriptions.

Impotence and Hypoglycemia

Reactive hypoglycemia, discussed in greater detail in chapter 3 (see p. 62), can be a cause of male impotence, even in young men. According to Cheraskin and Ringsdorf (1976 p. 117), a study at the Tel Aviv Medical School in Israel, shows that abnormal carbohydrate metabolism must be reversed to treat impotent men. For this reason the basic dietary rules already laid down in earlier chapters make good sense for continued virility. That is, be sure you are eating whole grains (instead of refined flour and rice), fruit (instead of sugar), high-protein foods, no inordinate quantity of sweets, caffeine, or alcohol, and also take the trace minerals which are known to regulate carbohydrate metabolism—chromium, manganese, and zinc. Foods rich in chromium include brewer's yeast, clams, corn oil, and whole-grain cereals. Manganese-rich foods are bananas, bran, celery, cereals, egg yolks, leafy greens, legumes, liver, nuts, pineapples, and whole grains. We will be discussing zinc, and dietary sources of this critical mineral, later in this chapter.

Lead and Phosphorus

Kunin (1980) describes a strong connection between nutritional imbalances and sexual failure. Many American POWs who survived the Bataan Death March in 1942, complained primarily of their inability to maintain an erection following their severe starvation under their captors. (Many lost half their normal body weight!) Other sexual changes were also seen such as enlarged breasts and shriveled genitals. The men feared they were turning into eunuchs.

After adequate nutritional therapy these sexual problems were reversed. The cause seems to be related to the fact that during this period of intense starvation toxic heavy metals, especially lead, were released from the prisoners' bones, bringing about impotence. Such lead mobilization can be reversed by using ample phosphorus in the diet (Kunin 1980, p. 154). This mineral, found in abundance in fish, eggs, milk, nuts, seeds, and beans, is an integral part of numerous sex hormones.

As one writer on aphrodisiacs tells the story, phosphorus will bring about severe male arousal; "but," he reports, "it's too easy to overdose oneself to death this way." We learn from the same writer that John Davenport, who wrote the first "full-length study of aphrodisiacs in English, tells the tale of a pharmacist's pet drake who drank water out of a vessel in which phosphorus had previously been kept and 'ceased not gallanting his females till he died (Selden 1979).' "

For the same reason that the POWs were impotent—a lack of phosphorus which allowed lead to enter the bloodstream from the bones—many men on crash diets also go through periods of impotence. To prevent this manifestation of lead toxicity extra quantities of iron, zinc, and vitamin C are crucial.

Zinc, Insanity, and Sperm

The old wives' tale about masturbation bringing about insanity has a possible link with current knowledge in nutritional science. Dr. Carl Pfeiffer of the Brain Bio Center in Princeton, New Jersey, explains that about two or more milligrams of zinc is lost during extended intercourse (Pfeiffer 1975, p. 471). Some men are very active sexually, or masturbate to excess, and also eat diets inadequate in this critical trace metal, which is utilized in the creation of sperm, seminal fluid, and many hormones. Such loss in an already zinc-depleted male could possibly produce psychological symptoms, as Dr. Pfeiffer observes:

> Perhaps with zinc-deficient males some degree of nervousness and even psychosis might result from excessive masturbation, but since the female loses little by way of secretions with masturbation, the old nineteenth century diagnosis of masturbatory insanity could scarcely be applied accurately to women.
>
> (Pfeiffer 1975, p. 471)

Even if you don't fear insanity it's a good idea to take extra zinc because most of our soils are depleted of this trace metal. The best food sources are oysters, shellfish, fish, whole grains (especially oatmeal), eggs, legumes, and nuts. Pumpkin seeds are particularly zinc-rich and are recommended regularly by European physicians who know that prostatitis can be controlled or reversed with zinc. Be sure that your vitamin/mineral pill contains at least thirty milligrams, or else supplement with a separate zinc tablet.

More on the Prostate

Few are the men who escape their fifties or sixties without some prostate trouble. Inevitably surgery ends the struggle, with the troublesome gland removed altogether, leaving behind a man not altogether what he once was in the sexual department.

This trouble can be avoided by following simple rules of preventive nutrition, including adequate amounts of zinc, from foods or supplements.

Dr. William R. Fair, chairman of Urology at Washington University in St. Louis, recently identified zinc as an antibacterial component in prostatic fluid (Fair 1977). He suggests that the trace metal acts to defend against chronic bacterial prostatitis and the urinary tract infections which follow. The fluid found in the prostate gland contains more of this metal than any other of our secretions or tissues! Moreover, the ability of our body to defend against infections in the prostate is directly correlated with the total zinc concentration in our prostatic fluid and semen.

Fair and co-workers examined the prostatic fluid from 15 men who suffered from chronic bacterial prostatitis. Remarkably, they discovered a depressed average zinc content of 50 micrograms per milliliter, as compared with an average 448 micrograms/milliliter zinc concentration in specimens taken from 49 healthy men!

It is important to remember that zinc inhibits cell division of invading bacteria *only in the presence of magnesium*. These two metals work together. For some good sources of magnesium, see Table A.3 in the Appendix.

In addition to greatly boosting your defenses against prostatitis, added zinc will speed wound healing, generally keep your immune system at a high level of preparedness, and greatly improve your senses of taste and smell, common functional losses with age. Just be sure to limit your overall zinc intake to under 100 milligrams from all sources. Too much can cause a sudden loss of iron from the liver, followed by a copper loss and the development of anemia.

Other Links in the Puzzle

Now, there are many other links between nutrients, sterility, and impotence. The evidence is not quite as solid as it is with the topics we have already discussed (carbohydrate metabolism, phosphorus, zinc, and magnesium), but they are still worth noting.

The B complex vitamins, in addition to playing a role in helping us cope with stress, are important in the maintenance of a healthy sex life. Pantothenic acid is critical to the formation of numerous hormones, while a pyridoxine (B_6) deficiency can lead to impotence. According to Pfeiffer (1975), deficiencies of vitamin B_6 and zinc are the most common cause of impotence in young men and amenorrhea in women.

It would be risky to leave this little review of men's problems and their nutritional cures without talking about vitamin E, since so many of you probably take this vitamin owing to its reputed value in maintaining healthy sperm. We don't want to knock this "sex vitamin," but it is overrated, at least for the male pursuit of virility. Now it is true, as the vitamin's discoverers found in the 1920s, that a lack of vitamin E causes rats to become sterile. It *is* essential in the functions of the gonads, and it *does* stimulate the production and motility of sperm (and also helps prevent miscarriages and premature births in pregnant females). But this is also true of other nutrients, and vitamin E must be part of an overall nutritional program, not viewed or taken as a sexual "upper." Wheat germ oil, eggs, leafy greens, nuts, and seeds, are all good sources. And, as you may remember from chapter 4 (on exercise), if you have diabetes, heart damage, or hypertension, vitamin E supplements can cause a severe and dangerous rise in blood pressure.

Oh yes, since we promised that this chapter is *"not for men only,"* Dr. Carl Pfeiffer suggests that folic acid be taken to elevate blood and tissue histamine levels in low-histamine women. It will provide easier orgasm.

Building Block #7:

"(Not) for Men Only:"
Your Protective Factors for Virility

Maintains balanced carbohydrate metabolism (See p. 114)	Assures adequate zinc intake from foods, supplements (See pp. 115)	Does not use recreational euphoriants
10 points	9 points	8 points
Takes vitamin E (See p. 117)	Takes vitamin B complex (See p. 117)	Takes vitamin B_6 (See p. 117)
7 points	6 points	5 points
Drinks moderately (See p. 114)	Heavy metals deleted (See p. 114)	Eats magnesium-rich foods (See p. 114)
4 points	3 points	2 points

Total the points for your present   Your Score
protective factors.   Block #7 _____

To page 139

for your next building block

8

ALONG THE ALIMENTARY CANAL:

Overcoming Constipation and its Attendant Ills

The Modern Plague of Constipation

Prehistoric stools show no signs of constipation. A few years ago we visited a parasitology laboratory at the University of California at Berkeley, to learn what nutritional knowledge can be gained from the study of coprolites, or fossilized remains of human feces. Standing transfixed before a bell jar which contained an ancient bowel movement, we watched it being *re*hydrated, to its original size, right before our eyes. Two things struck us. First, we were awed by the tremendous age of this specimen. Second, we were impressed by its large *size*. What was the secret of our long-extinct ancestors, that they were capable of such exuberant bowel movements?

We might imagine an anthropologist of the future looking for clues about our civilization by viewing old videotapes of commercial television programming. What conclusions might this scholar of a millennium hence draw from our proliferating advertisements for constipation remedies? What ails our civilization that we must be so preoccupied with our bowel movements, or lack thereof?

Unfortunately, many "enlightened" contemporary medical authorities tell us not to worry about constipation—that it's the worry itself that is doing the damage, not the plugging up of our bowels. We must respectfully disagree with this point of view. Just as it's normal to eat every day, so should it be normal to excrete waste and the undigested residue of our diet on an equally regular daily basis. And constipation doesn't *feel* right; you should be able to trust your body when it tells us that.

Many constipation remedies can be harmful. Constipation was *not* discovered in the latter half of the twentieth century, although it was only recently recognized as a chronic problem. Our grandparents had all sorts of cures for the condition, ranging from shockingly effective (and sometimes harmful) cathartics, to mechanical procedures such as colonic irrigation. These "colonics" generally faded out of favor as the pharmaceutical industry came up with a whole new line of laxative preparations to supplement the old folk remedies.

But none of these solutions is really ideal. Americans spend millions upon millions of dollars a year on laxatives, both prescription drugs and over-the-counter preparations. Many of these can be damaging to the bowel, desensitizing the nerves that activate peristalsis, disturbing the acid-base balance in the gut, and overstimulating the glands that secrete the digestive enzymes as they try desperately to protect the intestinal mucosa from these irritating substances. Mineral oil, an old remedy which is still used today, interferes with the absorption of vitamin A from our food. And, now that colonic irrigation has come back into vogue among some "holistic" practitioners, we must warn that this procedure can be equally harmful. When the contents of the bowel are excessively liquefied, the toxic substances in the stool are more readily absorbed through the walls of the intestine into the bloodstream. The protective mucous secretions are washed away; and the nerves, constantly subjected to the mechanical irritation of washing, may lose their ability to respond to the stimulus of stool present in the intestines.

In search of the "ideal" bowel movement. Although current medical wisdom tends to play down the dangers of constipation, there is very good evidence that this common problem may lie at the root of many of our modern illnesses. What is the ideal frequency and character of normal bowel elimination? Let's get downright graphic for a moment. The ideal bowel movement that we are all striving (though hopefully not straining) for, should be *large, soft, and frequent*. Once a day is a reasonable goal. The hard, dry, infrequent stools so common among us, if they become chronic, are just the first warning signs of bigger trouble ahead.

What Happens in the Colon Affects the Whole Body

Nutritional thinking often focuses on the stomach and small intestines as the "business end" of the digestive process. It's in the twenty-three odd feet of small intestine that most of our food is broken down by enzymes into the nutrients we require to rebuild, repair, and nourish our body's cells and to provide the fuel for our cellular energy processes. After all this chemical activity has transpired in the small intestine, the indigestible residue from our food passes on into the large intestine, or colon. At this point the fecal mass is half liquid, half solid in form. The solid material leads the way, stimulating the muscular walls of the colon to contract behind the mass, pushing it along, while the excess water is soaked up through the intestinal walls.

The colon is the home for large quantities of bacteria, which under healthy, balanced conditions are responsible for such important functions as manufacturing vitamin K, biotin, and other B vitamins. In fact, as much as thirty percent of the stool that is eventually excreted consists of bacteria!

What happens in the colon also affects the digestive process back upstream in the small intestine. Our body operates through many complicated biochemical feedback systems, and what transpires in the colon can trigger responses in the liver—affecting the secretion of bile and the conversion of cholesterol into bile.

All these processes depend, of course, on the fecal

mass moving through the colon at the proper rate and in
the proper, semiliquid form. If anything happens to slow
down or arrest that movement, many things can go wrong.
The bacterial population may change from beneficial to
harmful forms; the liver may begin to get improper signals;
the fecal mass may become hard and dry, irritating the
intestinal walls and pressing on the blood vessels that
supply nutrition to these tissues; the mucosal lining may
become irritated; and dangerous, toxic substances may
begin to collect in the colon, potentially damaging the
intestinal mucosa. All these highly undesirable consequences
can result from constipation. It's no wonder we instinc-
tively wish to avoid this condition!

Fiber as a Protective Factor

If you've been reading the health-oriented literature
over the past decade, you already know the answer to the
collective dilemma of our constipated modern civilization.
Over the past century there has been a radical change in
the nature of our food. Something very important has
been removed—something that was once thought to have
no importance in nutrition, but that is now recognized as
being an important constituent of the diet. That missing
something is fiber.

Fiber is a collective term describing hundreds of different carbohydrate-based compounds that occur naturally
in the vegetable kingdom. This is the material that our
grandmothers used to refer to as roughage. Fiber provides
the supporting structure in the leaves, fruit, and stems of
plants.

Originally the plant fiber in our food was known as
crude fiber, which was defined as the residue that re-
mained after plant material had been treated with acid and
alkali in the laboratory. However, this chemical process
measures only part of the fiber that is actually usable by
the human body. In 1972 the more useful concept of
dietary fiber was introduced. Dietary fiber refers to plant
materials that are not broken down by human digestive
enzymes. The most common form of fiber is cellulose;

other important kinds are hemicellulose, lignin, pectin, gums, and mucilages. These materials vary somewhat in their effects in the human digestive system and throughout the body, as we shall see later.

Fiber is lost in milling of grain. The fiber began to disappear significantly from our food at the time that the food-processing industry began to mill grains to produce the familiar white, powdery flour that has become the bane of today's nutritionists. Up until about 1880 most grain was stone-ground, leaving the healthful germ and bran in the whole-grain flour. With the introduction of steel milling, not only were most vitamins and minerals removed from the grain, but most fiber as well. The major part of this fiber occurred in the bran, the outer coating of the grain. At the turn of this century the average American consumed about 225 pounds of flour a year, half of which was whole wheat. Today, the average American eats only about 111 pounds of flour, and of that amount 104 pounds are white flour! Since white flour contains only 8 percent of the fiber found in whole wheat flour, it is obvious where the fiber content of our diets has disappeared to.

Fruits and vegetables a source of fiber. Add to that statistic a corresponding change in the way we consume fruits and vegetables, another important source of dietary fiber. The fiber content of these nutritious foods is largely destroyed or removed through processing—the removal of peels, excessive cooking, and various preserving and freezing methods. Our consumption of *processed* fruits and vegetables has more than doubled over the past 50 years, while our intake of these foods in their fresh, high-fiber state has been cut in half. Thus, while our overall consumption of fruits and vegetables has actually *increased* during this century, the widespread use of processed foods has led to a net *decrease* in the intake of fiber—as well as other important nutrients.

How High-Fiber Native Diets Protect Against Many Ills

The connection between the processing of foods and the change in the nature of bowel movements was first discovered by British doctors working with native villagers in Africa. These doctors noted that there was a distinct difference between the size and frequency of the natives' stools and those of Englishmen. The food eaten by the Africans moved along through their digestive tracts at a respectable clip, ending up in the stool in about 24 hours, whereas in Englishmen, the food might hang around in the intestines for three days before being excreted, and some Britishers would take as long as two weeks to process their food!

The British doctors found the explanation for this striking difference when they looked at the diets eaten by the two groups. They noted that the African villagers ate completely unprocessed, natural diets rich in unprocessed grains—diets containing high-fiber content. Their English patients, on the other hand, were eating typically "Western" foods: refined white flour, sugar, and fat. Whereas the African villagers were eating some 25 grams of fiber a day, the British (and we Americans as well) consume only about 8 grams of fiber a day.

The British doctors made an even more startling discovery. Not only were the Africans free of that plague of modern civilization, constipation, but they were also virtually free of many diseases that have come to be accepted as common in the modern world—coronary heart disease, cancer of the colon and rectum, appendicitis, hemorrhoids, diverticulosis and diverticulitis, varicose veins, phlebitis, and obesity!

While the Englishman Denis Burkitt was largely responsible for bringing the message about dietary fiber to the modern Western nations, it is important that we pay homage to an early worker in the field, whom we may consider Burkitt's guru. This brilliant scientist T. L. Cleave, is largely unknown in medical circles today; but his early paper, "The Neglect of Natural Principles in Current Medical Practice," published in 1956, provided the inspiration

for much subsequent research. We would like to quote
Burkitt in his testimony to this earlier worker's genius:

> When Cleave formulated his ingenious hypothesis link-
> ing many diseases characteristic of economic develop-
> ment to the refining of carbohydrate foods, he unwit-
> tingly threw light on the possible etiology of the malig-
> nancy responsible for more deaths than any other in
> the Western world except for bronchial carcinoma [i.e.,
> cancer of the colon and rectum—now the *most* com-
> mon form of fatal cancer!]. He recognized that some
> conditions characteristic of the more affluent com-
> munities, including atherosclerosis, obesity, dental
> caries, diabetes, diverticular disease, appendicitis, and
> varicose veins only became common after Western
> patterns of diet were adopted. Since the major dietary
> changes in the more economically developed countries
> during the period in which these diseases have be-
> come common concern the carbohydrate rather than
> the fat or protein fractions of food he sought an explana-
> tion for the diseases associated geographically and chron-
> ologically with changes made in carbohydrate foods.
> The massive refining of carbohydrates, a change intro-
> duced in Europe and North America mainly during
> the final quarter of the last century, seemed to him a
> likely factor. He considered the refining of sugar with
> almost total removal of fiber and protein from the
> natural product the chief cause, but also took into
> account the replacement of whole meal by refined
> flour. The diminished consumption of other high-fiber-
> content foods such as oatmeal and vegetables must also
> be considered.
>
> These "Western" diseases are certainly associated
> geographically and in many instances tend to be re-
> lated to one another in individual patients; my epide-
> miological studies in Africa and elsewhere substantiate
> Cleave's basic hypothesis.
>
> Changes made in carbohydrate foods may of course
> be only one of many etiological factors, but in some
> instances they would appear to be the major one.
>
> (Burkitt 1971, p. 916)

Now, as Burkitt acknowledges, it would be overly
simplistic to attribute *all* the difference in disease inci-

dence to the difference in fiber intake. Most likely the
Africans were partly protected against these diseases by
higher levels of physical activity, and possibly by freedom
from the kind of stress that is now recognized to be a
contributing factor in many "diseases of civilization." But
the role of diet was clearly important, as was demonstrated by the fact that as native African villagers moved to
the cities or migrated to Western nations, giving up their
traditional high-fiber diets for the highly processed "civilized" foods of the Western world, they began to develop
these same diseases—not immediately, but after an inter-
val that showed that it takes time for fiber deficiency to
take its toll on the body.

These facts were further supported by studies showing that Japanese who abandoned their traditional high-
fiber diets, either in Japan or on moving to Hawaii, also
showed an increased incidence of these "diseases of civilization." Moreover, in the Western world these diseases only
began to appear in significant proportions after overly
processed grains became a part of the diet.

The Fiber Connection in Common Diseases

Just what is it about fiber that helps to prevent constipation and to protect us against such a wide assortment of
diseases as cancer of the colon, heart disease, diverticulosis,
and all the rest? First of all, the fiber in our diet adds
significant bulk to our stools, providing more of a stimulus
to the ring-shaped muscles of the colon to contract behind
the fecal mass and push it along. Secondly, fiber has the
ability to absorb large quantities of water, helping to keep
the stool softer and preventing it from drying out as it
gives up its liquid contents to the mucosal walls of the
colon. The overall effect of the increased stool bulk and its
softness is to keep it moving, so that it is excreted promptly
before it has a chance to become hard and dry from
overlong retention in the colon.

Thus, through the simple mechanical properties of
fiber, we are protected significantly from the discomfort
and dangers of constipation. In addition, some diseases

that probably have their start with constipation are also significantly reduced in people who consume a high-fiber diet. Dr. David Reuben, in *The Save Your Life Diet* (1975), has clearly explained for us the connection between low fiber and a host of modern diseases.

Diverticulosis. A very common disease of the colon, diverticulosis occurs in some forty percent of Americans over the age of forty, although not always diagnosed as such. The condition is the result of increased internal pressure in the colon, caused by hard, dry stool that moves along too slowly, so that the walls of the colon shrink down. At weak points along the walls of the colon (generally surrounding blood vessels) little balloonlike bulges begin to form, known as diverticula. Hard plugs of fecal matter may get trapped in these little balloonlike diverticula, leading to inflammation and infection, which is the beginning of the much more serious condition known as diverticulitis.

People who eat a high-fiber diet are much less likely to develop diverticulosis and its related conditions than are low-fiber eaters. Diverticulosis wasn't even recognized as a disease in Western medical literature until about 1920—further evidence that it was the historical process of the overmilling of grains and the removal of the fiber from our food supply that was responsible for the development of this modern disease.

Appendicitis. Once we understand the mechanics of the large bowel, it is easy to see how other medical problems, such as appendicitis, can also develop with a low-fiber diet. Appendicitis can be a life-threatening condition, and some 200,000 appendectomies are performed each year. While it isn't entirely clear how appendicitis develops, constipation is probably a contributing factor.

The appendix is a short, dead-end tube about two and a half inches long, which opens off the point where the small and the large intestines meet. When the feces move too slowly through the intestine, they become hard and dry, and small fecaliths, or "fecal stones," may block the opening that leads into the appendix, closing it off and encouraging the development of infection. Changes in the bacterial population of the intestines may also contribute to appendicitis; we will be discussing the important role of bacteria.

No matter what is the exact cause of appendicitis, all the evidence seems to indicate that in the presence of a high-fiber diet the incidence of the disease drops markedly. Unlike the other medical conditions associated with low-fiber intake, such as diverticulosis and colon cancer, which show up toward middle age, appendicitis can also affect children. Similarly, the historical pattern indicates that when food processing removes fiber from a population's diet, appendicitis begins to occur in that population much earlier than the other low-fiber-related diseases.

Bacterial changes and colon cancer. Another significant change that takes place in the colon with a high-refined-carbohydrate, low-fiber diet is that the normally beneficial bacteria that inhabit the intestine, including *Streptococcus* and *Lactobacillus*, are replaced by another group of bacteria such as the *Bacteroides* and *Clostridium* species. Whereas the first group of bacteria are aerobic—that is, they thrive in an oxygen-rich environment—the latter, harmful group are anaerobic, requiring an oxygen-free environment. These anaerobic bacteria have the ability to break down the bile acids, secreted by the liver for the digestion of fats, into extremely dangerous cancer-causing substances. These carcinogens are most likely responsible for the high incidence of cancer of the colon among low-fiber-eating populations; in fact, cancer of the colon and the rectum is now the number one killer among all forms of cancer in the United States.

Of course, the dangers of the carcinogens in the colon would be reduced if the stool were excreted rapidly; but with people who eat low-fiber foods, the opposite is the case. Rather than moving through the bowel and carrying these harmful substances along, the slow-moving stool keeps these carcinogens in contact with the walls of the colon for inordinately long periods of time, perhaps up to seventy-two hours or more, giving them the opportunity to do their cancer-inducing work.

Heart disease and cholesterol control. Dietary fiber has also been shown to be related to the incidence of cardiovascular disease, the number one killer in this country.

We are all familiar today with the relationship between elevated levels of cholesterol in the bloodstream and the increased likelihood of fatal heart attacks. Cholesterol is not necessarily a harmful substance, and it plays a role in many normal metabolic processes in the body. Under normal conditions the liver converts some blood cholesterol into bile acids for the digestion of fats. Additional cholesterol is removed from the body through the colon when the stool is excreted, and so normal, regular bowel movements help to regulate the blood cholesterol level.

But when the harmful, anaerobic bacteria take over the colon in the presence of a low-fiber diet, the usual mechanism for converting blood cholesterol into bile acids is disrupted. One of the by-products of the breakdown of bile acids by these anaerobic bacteria is the compound lithocholate, which feeds back to the liver, telling it to stop converting cholesterol into bile acids. Thus, through both mechanical and chemical biofeedback mechanisms, the constipated colon contributes to elevated blood cholesterol levels. It is no surprise, then, that coronary disease was virtually unknown in medical literature at the beginning of this century. It is still extremely rare today among African villagers who continue to eat their traditional high-fiber diets.

Hemorrhoids. It isn't difficult to imagine why a high-fiber diet helps to prevent hemorrhoids. Straining at stool produces a buildup of pressure in the colon and the associated blood vessels. Furthermore, hard, dry stool exerts harmful pressure on the walls of the colon and the veins supplying this part of the body. Both these factors probably contribute to the development of hemorrhoids—the painful, bulging, bleeding veins around the anus with which too many Americans are familiar. Predictably, Africans and Asians who eat a high-fiber diet are essentially free of hemorrhoids. Their high roughage intake is likely part of the reason, although some workers have speculated that it is also because they squat to move their bowels rather than sit for prolonged periods of time on the toilet as we sedentary Westerners do.

Enthusiasts for the benefits of fiber extend the list of fiber-related diseases even further. They say that *varicose veins* are aggravated by low-fiber intake and that adequate fiber in the diet will help prevent the dangerous allied conditions of *thrombophlebitis* and *embolism*. Even *obesity* may be partly due to the low-roughage diet—not only because our modern diet contains so many "empty calories" that put on pounds without satisfying our appetite or nourishing us, but also because the actual absorption of calories may be reduced through the addition of fiber to the diet.

The Fiber Craze Hits the Supermarkets

When the benefits of dietary fiber were first pro-pounded in the health literature, a predictable thing happened. Everyone hurried off to buy high-fiber cereals, high-fiber breads, and other foods that were rushed to market to satisfy the new fiber craze.

But, as with most matters of nutrition, things aren't as simple as they may at first appear. Of course the most obvious thing would have been to return to high-fiber foods such as whole grains, fresh fruits, and vegetables. But the food-processing industry, which had removed the fiber from our food in the first place, found a much more complicated—and profitable—solution. If you look on your supermarket shelves today, you may find certain brands of high-fiber bread proudly proclaiming on their labels that they contain alpha-cellulose. Now, alpha-cellulose is nothing but ground-up wood—*sawdust*—in a colorless, tasteless, crystalline form!

Even more seductive than sawdust was the call of the formerly lowly bran. Bran is the outer coating milled out of whole grains. It happens that bran has the highest fiber content of any natural food, and so people began shoveling down mouthfuls of the dry, somewhat woody-tasting stuff, adding it to everything from their breakfast cereal to their ice cream, or stirring it into their orange juice.

Phytates a danger in bran. But, as is often the case with simplistic solutions, there's a catch. Unfortunately, bran contains substances known as phytates. Derived from the phosphorus compound phytic acid, phytates have the ability to interfere with the absorption of important mineral nutrients such as zinc, iron, and calcium, as well as other critical trace elements such as manganese, copper, and magnesium. Excessive consumption of phytates can lead to actual *deficiencies* of these important nutrients, and for this reason we must be cautious about consuming bran and other phytate-rich foods in excessive quantities.

Table 8.1 will help you to identify the phytate content of various fiber-rich foods. The foods on the left-hand side of the table are *low* in phytates, while those on the right have *high* phytate levels. By eating more of the fiber-rich foods toward the left side of the list you will ensure a high-fiber intake without the risks of excessive phytates.

Be cautious, also, concerning the bran cereals that are so widely sold today. Not only may there be excessive phytates in these cereals, but many of them also contain added sugar—the most refined, and most harmful, of carbohydrates.

Table 8.1

Phytate Levels in Fiber-Rich Foods

No Phytate	Traces of Phytate Levels	Moderate Phytate	Higher Phytate Levels
Celery	Broccoli	Artichokes	Cereals
Lettuce	Carrots	Potatoes	Legumes
Mushrooms	Green Beans	Sweet Potatoes	Nuts
Onions			
Spinach	Blackberries		
Apples	Figs		
Bananas	Strawberries		
Citrus fruits			
Pineapples			
Prunes			

Restoring Fiber to the Diet the Natural Way

We have already mentioned that the average American eats about 8 grams of fiber a day, and that the native

African eats some 25 grams. For most people, an intake of
about 20 grams of fiber per day should be a realistic goal,
sufficient to protect our health and guard against constipation and all the other diseases associated with low-fiber
intake. How can we guarantee this beneficial minimum
level of fiber intake without eating sawdust or swallowing
mouthfuls of phytate-loaded bran?

Fresh fruits and vegetables confer many benefits. The
solution lies along already familiar lines. The first step is to
return to a more natural way of eating, avoiding highly
processed foods, refined carbohydrates, white flour, and
white sugar, and instead eating plenty of fiber-rich fresh
fruits and vegetables, whole grains, nuts, seeds, and
legumes. All these foods are high in fiber and also provide
beneficial vitamins and minerals. At the same time, most
Americans should shift the balance of foods on their plate,
cutting back significantly on their intake of meats and
depending for some of their protein on a carefully thought
out balance of whole grains, legumes, and other protein-
rich plant foods.

When you eat fresh fruits and vegetables, don't throw
away the peels. They contain much of the fiber in these
foods. And, whenever possible, eat the seeds and cores as
well. Cook potatoes in their skins, which are a valuable
source of fiber. Eat vegetables raw or lightly steamed for
maximum nutritional benefits.

Many ethnic dishes use high-fiber foods, such as bulgur
wheat, kasha, corn tortillas, and whole wheat pasta. Remember that most processed snack foods are low in fiber
just as they are high in fat, sugar, salt, and possibly
harmful additives, while fresh fruits, nuts, seeds, and
unbuttered popcorn all make for nutritious, high-fiber
snacks.

In short, let the fiber in your diet be included as a
natural constituent of your food rather than gulping it down
as a separate supplement.

Leavened bread has reduced phytates. The disadvan-
tages of phytates can be partially overcome by using whole
grains and bran to make bread. During breadmaking,
yeast releases an enzyme known as phytase which breaks
down the phytic acid. In order to encourage the activity of

phytase, let your bread dough rise two or even three times. Making your dough acid, through the use of molasses, yogurt, sour milk, or fruit juice, will also encourage phytase to break down phytic acid (Robertson, Flinders, and Godfrey 1978, pp. 495–96).

Our intestines also contain phytase for breaking up phytic acid compounds. Remember that whole populations in many parts of the world live on phytate-loaded whole grain products and legumes without developing the mineral deficiencies that would arise without compensating mechanisms. In the case of calcium, one of the minerals affected by dietary phytates, we know that vitamin D helps our bodies to use this mineral efficiently, so sunshine and perhaps vitamin D supplementation will help to protect against calcium deficiencies.

Different fibers have different benefits. Remember, also, that dietary fibers from different sources differ not only in their chemical and physical properties, but in their effects on the body as well. Cereal bran and other sources of cellulose have a much greater effect on the size and transit time of stool than do the fibers from fruits and vegetables. Fibers from fruits and vegetables, such as pectin, gum guar, carrageenan, and others, have a cholesterol-reducing property, while the cellulose fibers are not active in this regard. Thus you should be careful to eat a *variety* of fibers in order to benefit from their combined protective effects. Someday it may be possible to determine specific needs for specific types of fiber sources, depending on the physiological needs of the individual.

Fiber Counting: A New Way to Design Your Diet

The "partial menus" in Table 8.2 will show you several ways to reach the goal of at least 20 grams of fiber intake per day. Just be sure to include these or *other* like foods *with your regular diet*. By referring to Table 8.3, you can see how easy it is to get the "fiber habit." You will not only facilitate bowel regularity, but also gain the vitamins and minerals so intimately connected with high-fiber *whole* foods. As an added plus you will probably see your serum cholesterol and triglyceride levels fall dramatically, after a few months.

Table 8.2

How To Get 20 Grams of Fiber a Day by Adding Simple Foods to Your Diet*

Meal (Use these or *other* like foods* with your regular diet)	Fiber Content
Breakfast:	
1 banana	2 gm.
⅔-cut whole wheat/corn or barley flakes	3 gm.
1 slice whole wheat bread	2 gm.
Lunch:	
2 slices whole wheat bread	4 gm.
1 orange	2 gm.
lettuce (on sandwich)	1 gm.
bean sprouts (on sandwich)	1 gm.
Dinner:	
1 baked potato with skin	4 gm.
1 stalk broccoli	3 gm.
baked beans, 2 tablespoons	2 gm.
Total Added Fiber for 3 Meals:	24 gm.
Snack Foods:	
figs, dried (3.5 oz.)	5.6 gm.
1 cup strawberries	4 gm.
almonds (3.5 oz.)	2.6 gm.
dates (3.5 oz.)	2.3 gm.
sesame seeds (1 oz.)	2 gm.

* See Table 8.3, "Other Fiber-Rich Foods to Add to Your Meals."

Table 8.3

Other Fiber-Rich Foods to Add to Your Meals*

Food	Grams of Fiber per 100 grams (100 gm. = 3½ oz.)	Food	Grams of Fiber per 100 grams (100 gm. = 3½ oz.)
Unprocessed bran	9.1	Pecans	2.3
All-Bran or Bran Buds	7.8	Prunes (dried)	2.2
Elderberries	7.0	Shredded Wheat Cereal	2.2
Sesame Seeds	6.3	Popcorn	2.2
Dried Figs	5.6	English Walnuts	2.1
Black Raspberries	5.1	Peanut Butter	1.9
Coconuts	4.0	Grape Nuts Flakes	1.8
Sunflower Seeds	3.8	Whole Wheat Bread	1.6
Kumquats	3.7	Grape Nuts	1.5
Bran Flakes Cereal	3.6	Green Peppers	1.4
Currants	3.4	Winter Squash	1.4
Brazil Nuts	3.1	Pumpkins	1.3
Filberts	3.0	Strawberries	1.3
Loganberries	3.0	Lentils	1.2
Peanuts	2.7	Pumpernickel Bread	1.1
Almonds	2.6	Turnips	1.0
Macadamia Nuts	2.5	Corn Flakes	0.7
Wheat Germ	2.5	Celery	0.6
Dates	2.3	Bananas	0.5

Source: *Saturday Evening Post* January 1977.

Adjusting to the high-fiber diet. Some people experience some uncomfortable symptoms when they first increase their fiber intake, largely because of the changes in the bowel bacteria. There may be an increase in gas, as evidenced by bloating or flatulence. This *may* be helped by taking live *Lactobacillus* culture, or *Acidophilus* milk products. In any case, as your digestive system adjusts to changed conditions—which are really *normal* conditions—the gassiness should abate.

Troubleshooting Your Constipation

Now that we've shown you that constipation can be a dangerous condition, and can lead to more serious diseases, it wouldn't be fair to tell you to eat lots of whole grains and fresh fruits and vegetables, and let it go at that. For many people this simply isn't going to be enough.

Some people will begin to experience the desired large, soft, and frequent bowel movements simply by adding fiber-rich foods to their diets. Others, however, may not see such immediate, gratifying results. What if you're doing everything right, eating all those fiber-rich grains, raw fruits, and vegetables until you feel like a walking salad, and you're still constipated? For stubborn cases, it may help to examine some additional factors.

Stress contributes to constipation. One possible explanation is that the trouble is in your head. Much as we've been emphasizing quite the opposite end of the anatomy, the fact remains that in our fast-paced modern civilization, emotional stress does take a significant toll, and one of the ways it can express itself is through a stoppage of normal peristaltic movements in the intestines. Constipation can also be a symptom of depression. If your constipation is long-standing, and you suspect psychological factors, consult your doctor for medical treatment until your corrected diet can begin to work for you.

Even better than taking medications is reducing stress or depression through exercise, meditation, or relaxation techniques. Passionflower herbal tea is an excellent substitute for tranquilizers. One teaspoonful of the dried herb, per cup of boiling water, *unsweetened,* will relax you *without* impeding your ability to think. This should let your body achieve its own "miracles" on a high-fiber diet.

Medications can cause constipation. Opiate painkillers such as codeine, iron preparations such as ferrous sulfate, some antacids, some diuretics, and certain tranquilizers, can all cause constipation. One very common cause of constipation is an excessive use of laxatives. Frequent watery stools deplete fluid and potassium and lead to a loss of muscular tone in the large intestine. The end result is a decreased urge to defecate. Incidentally, be sure to respond to the urge promptly when you feel it. Postponing your bowel movements will also produce constipation.

How foods may affect bowel function. If you've been making a serious effort to clean up your dietary act, your body may be going through a period of readjustment. Refined sugar, for instance, is notoriously laxative in its effects. Of course, with the regular intake of refined sugar our body adapts and doesn't necessarily respond with loose bowel movements; but if you've made an effort to eliminate sugar from your diet, your body may be readjusting to the sudden absence of this substance.

Wine and tea contain tannins. Tannin has the effect of drying out the mucous lining of the intestinal tract, and may be responsible for a drying and hardening of the stool. While you may need to cut back on your tea consumption, be sure to drink plenty of fluids, including a glass of water with each meal.

Some people find that nothing will stimulate a bowel movement like a piece of meat! While this may appear contrary to all the dietary wisdom we've related in this chapter, it is wise to bear in mind that *some* fat is essential and that man has always been an omnivore, eating animals as well as plants.

While we're on the subject of animal foods, let's not forget the "fibrous" portions of animal products. Bones, shells of seafood like shrimp, and insect shells were a part of early man's diet, and perhaps we still need these foods today. Although animal-derived "fiber" is broken down in the digestive process, unlike vegetable fiber, it may serve purposes that have not yet been identified—and it can also be an excellent source of calcium and other minerals that may be depleted through the consumption of phytate-rich bran and other foods. This is why we recommend that you eat the soft bones of chicken, fish, and other animals, along with the flesh.

Rate Your Protective Factors Against Constipation

It should be clear by now why it's so important for you to rate well on your intake of protective fiber-rich foods. Once you've begun increasing your fiber intake, go back and review the other building blocks in this book. You'll be amazed how your "protection scores" against many other diseases have also increased at the same time!

Building Block #8:

"Along the Alimentary Canal:"
Your Protective Factors Against Constipation

Fiber* intake is 25–30 grams a day or more (See p. 132) 35 points**	Fiber* intake is 20–24 grams a day (See p. 133) 25 points**	Fiber* intake is 15–19 grams a day (See p. 133) 16 points**
Fiber* intake is 10–14 grams a day (See p. 133) 8 points**	Rarely constipated (See p. 136) 7 points	Avoids excessive high-phytate fiber foods (See p. 130) 5 points
Handles stress without drugs (See p. 136) 4 points	Avoids laxatives (See pp. 136, 137) 3 points	Fiber* intake is 9 grams a day or less (See p. 133) 2 points**

Total the points for your present protective factors.**

Your Score
Block #8 _____

---

*Fiber refers to plant material from fresh food, *not* bran! (See p. 122)
**Score yourself for *only* the highest-value "fiber" square for which you qualify. The score for that square includes scores for all lower levels of fiber intake.

To page 171

for your next building block

9

NEGATIVE-CALORIE FOODS:*

Controlling Weight the Easy Way

People will go to desperate lengths in order to rid themselves of excess weight. Not that many years back, around the same time as the "Hollywood Diet" (pushed by the melba toast and grapefruit interests), many individuals submitted themselves to the "tapeworm cure" for obesity. In this treatment the patient swallowed a tablet containing an embryonic tapeworm that grew to take care of any extra food that was eaten!

But people did not stop at infesting themselves with parasites in order to get thin. Many imitated (and still do) the gluttons of ancient Rome by inducing vomiting after a meal, to rid themselves of the food.

Besides the repulsiveness of the "tapeworm cure," the "Roman glutton" method, and other drastic measures, there is a good deal of danger involved in these extremes. Not only is the body robbed of the nutrients it must have, but the organ systems become stressed, sometimes fatally. This is also true of high colonic irrigation, another attempt

---

*While this concept is negated by some workers in the field, it has been included as the weight-loss method of choice owing to the high-fiber, high-nutrient density of the suggested foods for this *limited* time of dieting.

140

to cheat nature in the pursuit of slenderness. Some doctors endorse two or three such drastic enemas daily. But this type of "irrigation" if repeated too frequently often irritates the bowel, resulting in intestinal inflammation while depriving the patient of essential nutrients.

Total fasting is also alien to the principles of this book. It may be an effective treatment for people with some chronic disorders, such as epilepsy, but is completely ineffective, in the long run, for overweight people. Why? Because the starvation method induces a sense of emotional loss so drastic that the weight lost during a crash fast is gained back in a few days when the overwrought individual inevitably goes on a food binge. Also, the depletion of most essential protective nutrients opens the way for possible disease states. Actually the overindulgence that always follows a total fast, whether it be one or two weeks later, is the body's way of replenishing the nutrients depleted during starvation. In this sense the eating binge is natural, however frustrating.

The weight loss plan we recommend is based on "negative-calorie" foods. These foods actually require more energy (that is, calories) to be metabolized than they yield. So you can eat as much of them as you want without gaining one net calorie! This dietary approach has satisfied many people because it is really a moderate fasting regimen with wine permitted, based upon ancient health and dietary ideas.

One of the first documented examples of a long-term modified fast, once widely quoted by dietitians, is that of Luigi Cornaro, an Italian nobleman of the Renaissance who lived to the ripe old age of 98. He attributed his longevity to the fact that he reduced his food consumption to a subsistence level. At the age of 40 Cornaro was a very sick man, given only a few months to live by his medical advisers. But he was determined not to die, and he set out to starve himself back to health. He succeeded so well that at the age of 95 he was mentally and physically sound, and able to work at his desk eight hours a day. Beginning at the age of 83, Cornaro wrote a series of essays entitled *Vita Sobria,* where he describes how he reduced his daily food intake to twelve ounces. But he also drank fourteen

ounces of wine every day. We have determined that he
averaged only 1,200 calories per day, and that during his
latter years, he managed to reduce still further the amount
he ate, but continued to drink his allotted quantity of
wine.

Known as the Centenarian's Diet, this modified fast
has been criticized by the medical establishment because
of a lack of corroborative evidence. But whether this man
actually ate only 1,200 calories is unimportant. His method
was excellent and worked principally because he did not
subject himself to an unlivable diet. He allowed himself
the pleasure of wine.

To lose the five to ten pounds of extra weight you
might gain from time to time during your middle years,
the "Negative-Calorie Diet" is your best approach. It is
not extreme, and should be followed for *two to three days*
at a time, alternating with the sensible dietary principles
laid down throughout this book.

The foods to eat, *raw* or steamed, are listed in Table
9.1.

Table 9.1

Negative-Calorie Foods
(Eat all you want and gain not one net calorie!)

Vegetables

Asparagus	Eggplant
Bean sprouts	Green pepper
Beets	Lettuce
Broccoli	Mushrooms
Celery	Summer squash
Carrots	Tomatoes
Cucumbers	

Fruits

Cantaloupe	Strawberries
Grapefruit	Watermelon

Notice that these are all *fiber*-rich, vitamin/mineral-
dense foods—exactly what you need to protect against

many of the diseases of aging. Of course, this diet is *not intended to be eaten on a daily basis*. It is deficient in protein, calories, calcium, and other nutrients required to sustain health on a long-term basis. However, for two- to three-day periods eating only these foods is an ideal way to keep your weight where you want it, or bring it back down to where it should be.

Drinking wine on this diet will help reduce the anxiety usually associated with a stressful starvation "no-fun" weight loss plan. One medium glass of dry white or red wine contains about eighty calories. We heartily recommend that you consider one such glass with each negative-calorie evening meal.

If you're the type who finds it hard to do just one of anything, mixing your glass of wine with mineral water is an excellent way to increase the pleasure but not the calories.

10

KEEPING YOUR MARBLES:

Nutrients for the Aging Brain

Senility Is Not Inevitable

When a 30-year-old mother, distracted by a telephone call, forgets to turn off the oven and overcooks the roast, she is called forgetful or scatterbrained. When a 70-year-old makes the same mistake, she is labeled senile, and perhaps a danger to herself and others. When a 40-year-old businessman suddenly experiences mental changes including confusion, his doctor rushes him through a complex workup, perhaps including such sophisticated studies as a CAT scan and cerebral arteriograms. When a 75-year-old retired executive comes into his doctor's office complaining of confusion, his doctor sends him home without treatment, diagnosing the problem as senility.

It is tragically true that many elderly people who are institutionalized with diagnoses of irreversible mental illness and senile dementia are in fact suffering, or were at first suffering, from such simple problems as nutritional deficiencies, adverse drug reactions, and other readily correctible disorders. Although the incidence of new psychiatric illness is higher among people over 65 than among any other age group (Butler 1975, p. 227), it is a mistake to assume that we must inevitably lose our memory, our mental acuity, and our sanity as we grow older. In fact, only a maximum of about 5 percent of our elder population are actually institutionalized for psychiatric problems, and of these only a small proportion suffer from the incurable senile dementia that so many people believe is an inevitable part of the aging process.

Normal aging does not produce senility; senile dementia is, properly speaking, a disease. But many problems with memory and cognition can arise from improper diet and unstimulating surroundings. And one of the best forms of insurance you can invest in to assure a healthy mind in your later years is to begin *right now* to eat a proper diet, making sure that you receive adequate quantities of key nutrients that have been shown to be linked with proper functioning of the brain.

Before we review these "mental nutrients," we need to take a closer look at what happens in the brain as the body ages.

The Aging Nervous System

From the moment we are born, our brains begin to lose nerve cells, or neurons. Unlike most other cells of the body, neurons don't reproduce; once a nerve cell dies, it will never be replaced. It has been estimated that the healthy brain of a young adult loses some 100,000 of its 12 billion neurons a day (Hoffer and Walker 1980, p. 17). But look at those figures: 12 billion is a lot of brain cells—more than we will ever use. Even at the rate of 100,000 cells lost a day, the brain has the capacity to remain functional right through very old age. On autopsies the brains of nonsenile, very old people may show shrinkage and the loss of perhaps 30 percent of the brain cells; yet, before these people died, they were healthy, alert, and functional.

Besides the decline in the absolute number of brain cells, the neurons undergo other changes with aging. Nerve fibers twist around each other to produce so-called neurofibrillary tangles. Other abnormal tissue accumulates, known as neuritic plaques. These plaques contain nerve fibers and a substance known as amyloid. All these changes take place as a part of the normal aging process, and tend to be concentrated in some parts of the brain more than others. Even with all these changes, however, most people do not suffer intellectual impairment. It is only when the plaques and tangles become abnormally profuse, especially in certain parts of the brain such as the hippocampus (the center of learning and memory), that senile dementia may occur.

Another change that occurs in the nerve cells is a reduction in dendritic branching. The dendrites are the fibers at the end of the nerve cells that transmit impulses from one neuron to another. Yet, recent research has suggested that even this loss of branching in the dendritic "tree" may be reversible under stimulating environmental conditions, as we will see later on.

It was formerly thought that all senile deterioration of mental functioning was the result of "hardening of the arteries of the brain." It is now recognized, however, that arteriosclerosis is *not* the principal cause of senile dementia. It is true that there are changes in the cerebral arteries with advancing age, but such changes apparently lead to decrements in mental functioning only when localized physical damage occurs, such as cerebral infarction, hemorrhages, or strokes. The survival of the nerve cells in the brain, and the brain's proper functioning, depend on a steady supply of oxygen, carried by the blood. It is obvious, then, that blockage of blood flow can cause irreversible damage to localized parts of the brain. When such damage is severe, or occurs in crucial areas, as in strokes, important losses in cognitive functioning may occur. (The prevention of strokes is largely related to the control of high blood pressure and the maintenance of a healthy circulatory system, and has been discussed in chapter 1.)

Among other changes in the aging brain is the accumulation of deposits of the brownish pigment lipofuscin. While some researchers have hypothesized that lipofuscin may "clog up" the cells, it is not known for certain whether this pigment is harmful or not. There is also a decrease in the levels of the brain hormone acetylcholine, the neurotransmitter that is involved in the transmission of nerve impulses and memory formation and storage. Changes in sleep patterns in the elderly, possibly partly due to neuron losses and structural changes of nerves in the brain's sleep center, may also contribute to changes in cognitive functioning.

The elderly brain is extremely sensitive to physical problems everywhere in the body. The brain may be the first, and often the only, organ to show signs of illness which in younger people might be manifested elsewhere. For example, among elderly heart attack victims, fifteen percent show no chest pains or other physical symptoms whatsoever, manifesting only confusion (Henig 1981, p. 88). Similarly, drug reactions, dehydration, renal failure, malnutrition, and a host of other problems, may produce symptoms in the elderly that look like senility, and if they are improperly diagnosed an elderly patient may be caught in a downward spiral of deteriorating health as unrecognized physical problems go untreated, dismissed as merely "senility."

Old People Aren't Stupid

It is now well established that most healthy old people remain as intelligent as they were when they were younger. In the past, many studies purported to show that intelligence test scores declined with age. However, these studies were *cross-sectional* in methodology, comparing the performance of a group of young subjects with that of older persons. Such studies failed to take into account the fact that the older people generally were less well educated than their youthful counterparts. Only relatively recently have large numbers of people received higher levels of education, and it has been well documented that education has a demonstrable effect on IQ scores. More recent studies have taken such differences into consideration, and it now appears that when a healthy, college-educated group of old people are compared with a healthy, well-educated younger group, their intellectual performance is comparable. While the elderly subjects may do slightly less well on certain tests such as spatial relations, they may actually do *better* than the younger subjects on numerical and verbal skills and inductive reasoning (Cherkin 1975, p. 179).

Similarly, it has been shown that healthy older people are just as capable of learning as younger people, and that, contrary to popular belief, they show no significant loss of memory function—either short-term or long-term—as compared with their juniors.

We have only to look at the many examples of older people who have produced great works of creative genius to realize that old age is not necessarily a time of intellectual decline. Frank Lloyd Wright produced his greatest architectural works after the age of 75; Michelangelo created the "Pieta" at 80; and Bertrand Russell was working on his autobiography at the age of 96.

One change in functioning that *does* occur with age is a slowing in reaction time, partly but not entirely due to a reduction in nerve transmission speed. This slowing may cause older people to do more poorly on tests that are scored according to speed of response, and may cause them to take longer to sift through their (larger) memory stores in search of the correct answer. But most elderly people, aware of the decline in their response speed, learn to compensate by striving for accuracy.

One factor that does have a very significant adverse effect on cognitive functioning is poor health. According to aging authority Butler (1975 p. 175), an estimated 86 percent of Americans over 65 have one or more chronic illnesses. It is obvious, then, that poor health may account for impaired intellectual functioning in a significant proportion of older people. Such diseases as high blood pressure and immune disorders have been shown to have a negative influence on intelligence test scores. Thus *it is health, not age itself, that is the most important determinant of cognitive functioning among the elderly*.

The Dangerous Myth of Senility

It is not only cruel to assume that people inevitably "go senile" when they grow old; it is also potentially very dangerous. Many changes in consciousness and memory may be symptoms of significant medical emergencies. When people assume that such mental changes in older people are "only senile symptoms," the medical emergencies go undiagnosed and untreated, and then the damage may become more extensive, perhaps leading to irreversible damage to mental and physical functioning.

For an unfortunate minority of elderly people, however, senile dementia is a real condition, characterized by memory loss, confusion, inability to perform simple problems in arithmetic, and disorientation as to time and place. While other, treatable causes can also produce such symptoms, in some cases they are due to irreversible destructive changes in the brain. Sometimes the damage is caused by localized blockage of the blood vessels, which cuts off the supply of vital oxygen to the tissues. In other cases the damage is to the nerve cells themselves, with an abnormally high concentration of plaques and tangles of nerve fibers, concentrated in specific areas of the brain. Such pathological changes in the brain cells, which can be positively diagnosed only on autopsies, are characteristic of the dreaded Alzheimer's disease. This form of senile dementia affects some 600,000 to one million Americans over 65, and perhaps another 60,000 or so who are younger. It is the fourth or fifth most common underlying cause of death in the nation (Henig 1981).

Fortunately, a reversible *nutritional* link has been uncovered. Canadian investigators have recently found aluminum at "above normal levels in the brains of some Alzheimer's patients postmortem" (Medical Tribune, April 28, 1982). While it is very difficult to achieve an aluminum free diet it is important that you greatly restrict your diet. Aluminum is added as an emulsifying agent to processed cheese (one slice may contain as much as two and a half times the average daily intake); in pickles it may appear as a firming agent; aluminum salts are added as a leavening agent to baking soda and cake mixtures; and tap water often contains added aluminum "to remove particulate matter." *Antacids* and *buffered* aspirins are notoriously high in aluminum. For example, 35–208 mg. of aluminum are found in a single anatacid tablet, and 10–52 mg. per aspirin tablet. (The average aluminum intake is about 20 mg./day.) In addition to all of these "pitfalls," cooking with aluminum pots may be as dangerous as the health-food "extremists" have said they are for many years, especially if the cooked food is allowed to sit.

In addition to being absorbed in the brain, it is thought that aluminum is deposited in the parathyroid gland and may lead to osteoporosis. This occurs because aluminum binds phosphorus in the gut, which will demineralize the bones. When combined with alcohol the situation is aggravated. Alcoholics who dose themselves with antacids greatly increase their risk of aluminum toxicity and associated diseases, including Alzheimer's.

What's the "cure" for this dread form of senility which can begin as early as age 40? Chelation using deferoxamine, "injected 21 consecutive days a month, for periods ranging from 4 to 24 months," has been tried experimentally with some success by Dr. Donald McLachlan, Professor of Physiology and Medicine at the University of Toronto.

Pseudosenility. Many cases of confusion and memory impairment in older people are not manifestations of senile dementia, but rather of so-called pseudosenility, a vague combination of complaints that can arise from any number of causes, most of them treatable. As psychiatrist Abram Hoffer observes, pseudosenility is one of the greatest hazards of growing old, for the consequences of being branded senile when you're not, can be fatal (Hoffer and Walker 1980, p. 45).

Psychiatrist Robert Butler won a Pulitzer prize for *Why Survive?* a study of the current status of the elderly in America. In this eye-opening book, Butler criticizes the routine way in which older people are dismissed as senile, leaving serious underlying conditions untreated:

> Chronic brain disorder is, of course, a reality for numbers of older people, but it has become a wastebasket diagnosis applied whenever anyone starts "acting senile."
>
> All too often, mentally confused older people are sent home untreated by doctors and hospitals when they are suffering from reversible confusional states—a sur-

prising number of which are due to malnutrition, anemia, alcohol and unrecognized physical ailments.

(Butler 1975, pp. 176, 226–27)

Some Causes of Pseudosenility

A wide variety of conditions can underlie the mental changes that are often mistaken for senility in the elderly. In general, the more rapid the onset of confusion and similar symptoms, the more likely they are due to a reversible problem.

Physical illness. In old people, any physical illness can produce an impairment in mental functioning. We have already mentioned that in many elderly people a heart attack may strike without chest pain, confusion being the only symptom. Changes in mental functioning may be the first, and sometimes the only, signs of a wide variety of disease conditions. Infection, anemia, gallstones, hepatitis, hypoglycemia, urinary retention—all these treatable problems and many others, can masquerade as senility.

Drug toxicity. Another very common cause of "reversible dementia" in the elderly is adverse reactions to drugs since their bodies are generally much more sensitive to medication than those of younger patients. The central nervous system is particularly sensitive to medications, especially those that have depressant effects. Physiological functions in the aging body are less efficient, with changes in kidney and liver function affecting the rate at which potentially toxic chemicals are removed from the body. Doctors must learn an entirely new set of rules in prescribing for the elderly patient, and dosages that may be safe and effective in younger adults can have damaging effects in older people. Thus many mental changes in elderly patients are directly traceable to iatrogenic, or treatment-induced, effects.*

The chance of iatrogenic effects is increased not only by the greater sensitivity of the elderly to medications, but also to the fact that older people generally take more

---

*Table 10.1, page 158, lists many psychological side effects for commonly prescribed drugs.

medications, and in greater combination, than younger people. For a variety of reasons, older people may not follow instructions properly. And, because many doctors are unaware of proper dosage levels for older patients and do not inquire what other drugs they may be taking, the doctor's instructions themselves are often wrong.

Endocrine and metabolic disorders. Glandular malfunction can also produce a form of confusion that is mistaken for "incurable" senility. Even mild hypothyroidism, or underactivity of the thyroid gland, can lead to mental changes in the elderly that look like senility. To make matters more confusing, even an *over*active thyroid in an old person can produce pseudosenility, whereas in younger people over- and underactive thyroids are readily distinguishable conditions, having opposite effects. Many elderly people manifesting confusion may simply be dehydrated, owing to an inadequate intake of liquids. Diminished thirst may in turn be due to a zinc deficiency.

Depression and other psychological disorders. Older people are at least as susceptible as younger people to depression and other psychiatric complaints. In younger people there would be little danger that depression would be mistaken for an irreversible brain syndrome; but older people are very often depressed and simply because of their age they are diagnosed as senile. As Robert Butler observes, emotional and mental disorders of old age are often not considered genuine mental illnesses:

> Some of what is called senile is the result of brain damage. But anxiety and depression are also frequently lumped within the same category of senility, even though they are treatable and often reversible. . . . It is all too easy to blame age and brain damage when accounting for the mental problems and emotional concerns of later life.
>
> (Butler 1975, p. 9)

Nutritional deficiencies. Of particular interest to this book are the many ways that nutritional deficiencies can produce the appearance of senility in the elderly. In a study by Dr. M. L. Mitra in an English hospital, it was found that the elderly suffer more severely from faulty diets than any other age group (Cheraskin and Ringsdorf 1976, p. 126). In many of Dr. Mitra's cases, mental confusion and disoriented behavior either diminished or disappeared after appropriate vitamin therapy was instituted.

Remember that as a nation the nutrition "density" of our diet has been deteriorating for decades. The older a person is, the longer has our overly refined and sugar-laden diet been able to take its toll on nutritional status. In fact, Dr. Abram Hoffer believes that many older persons have been deprived of important nutrients for so long that they can no longer be restored to proper nutritional status through food alone. In such cases of prolonged nutritional deficiencies, Hoffer believes that it is necessary to use megadoses of supplements in order to achieve adequate nutrition to the body's cells and to reverse the mental deterioration that is often an early symptom of chronic malnutrition:

> We believe that . . . deficiency of essential nutrients, when present for many decades in the form of subtle, chronic malnutrition, is the source of most premature aging and final senility. . . . These are aspects of aging and senility which have been almost totally ignored by establishment geriatricians.
>
> (Hoffer and Walker 1980, p. 66)

Changes in the functioning of the aging digestive system, and the reduction in appetite that may accompany old age, may have a further effect on the proper intake and utilization of essential nutrients. Added all together, dietary deficiencies can be one of the most significant factors in mental deterioration in the elderly.

Nutrients to Prevent or Reverse Senility

Certain specific nutrients are known to be associated with proper mental functioning. When adequate levels of these nutrients are lacking in the diet, the resulting deficiency states may include pronounced alterations in mental functioning, and when the nutrients are restored to the diet the mental symptoms are cured. In more recent years, it has been shown that very large doses of certain nutrients, particularly niacin, in conjunction with other B vitamins and vitamin C, have been able to cure not only classic deficiency diseases, but also such serious mental disorders as schizophrenia. In fact, orthomolecular medicine, or the use of very high doses of nutrients to treat illness, really had its start with the use of niacin by Hoffer and Osmond to treat schizophrenia.

Niacin. Niacin, or vitamin B_3, has proven the most useful in the treatment of failing memory and confusion that accompanies old age. One of the first documented uses of this vitamin to treat "senile" symptoms was a last-resort experiment by Dr. Abram Hoffer. Concerned by his mother's failing memory and vision at the age of 67, Hoffer tried giving her large doses of nicotinic acid (a form of niacin)—not because he really thought that the vitamin would be able to improve her memory, but because there was an outside chance that the recognizable flushing effect would produce a beneficial placebo response. To Hoffer's surprise and delight, his mother began to improve in her mental and physical functioning, and for 21 years she continued to take one to four grams of nicotinic acid a day, remaining mentally alert and active, even writing books, until she finally died following a stroke at the age of 87. While one case study hardly represents a scientific sample, we must not overlook the great analytical and intuitive abilities of a researcher of Dr. Hoffer's stature.

Hoffer recommends that any older person who shows depression, anxiety, confusion, and disorientation, should be treated with three grams a day of nicotinic acid; but it is far better, according to Hoffer, to begin nicotinic acid supplementation earlier in life, before there have been any irreversible changes in the brain or the nervous system's biochemistry. The earlier that an individual begins supplementation with nicotinic acid, the lower will be the dosage required. Hoffer suggests the following preventive dosage schedule:

Age 20–29	100 mg niacin after each meal
30–39	300 mg niacin after each meal

40–49	500 mg niacin after each meal
50 and over	1000 mg niacin after each meal
	(Hoffer and Walker 1980, p. 145)

The amide form of niacin, nicotinamide, or niacinamide, will not produce the sometimes unpleasant flushing that is characteristic of this vitamin, but Hoffer believes that older people will derive greater benefits from the nicotinic acid. The optimal dose in any case is that which effectively eliminates symptoms while producing minimal or no side effects.

Hoffer also reports that niacin has another important effect in that it appears to prevent "sludging" of the red blood cells. Red blood cells in some people have a tendency to stick together—the so-called rouleaux effect. Because they are clumped together, the red blood cells cannot travel freely through the tiny capillaries and carry vital oxygen to the tissues. Such oxygen starvation can obviously have severe effects on mental functioning. Many older people have sludging of the blood, and have a characteristic appearance of pale, puffy faces, along with fatigue, tension, and anxiety. When such people are treated with nicotinic acid, they are restored to their normal appearance and their red blood cells no longer clump together. Hoffer reports that anticoagulant drugs that help control sludging are helpful in treating senility, and that niacin is a significant antisludging substance, apparently working by increasing the negative electrical charge on the red blood cells so that they repel each other.

Other B vitamins. Other members of the B complex have also proven helpful in controlling mental problems that accompany aging. Thiamine deficiency, or beriberi, is known to produce psychiatric and neurological symptoms which might be mistaken for senile changes in an elderly person. A form of brain disease known as Wernicke-Korsakoff syndrome results from a partial destruction of the brain owing to the lack of thiamine; this condition is most commonly found in chronic alcoholics, but has been diagnosed in nonalcoholics as well. The symptoms are similar to those of senile dementia, with memory problems being the first to appear. The use of thiamine has been shown to reverse the clouded consciousness of Wernicke-Korsakoff syndrome in clinical studies (Cherkin 1975).

Since thiamine deficiency, or an increased need for thiamine, is the main cause of Wernicke-Korsakoff syndrome, Abram Hoffer suggests that thiamine be added to alcoholic beverages as a way of preventing the disease. A divided dosage of 250 milligrams a day is recommended. The consumption of large quantities of refined sugar can also produce a thiamine deficiency state, since thiamine is essential to sugar metabolism.

Another B vitamin, pantothenic acid, has been popularized by Dr. Roger Williams as an antiaging nutrient, and is required for the normal functioning of the nervous system.

To ensure adequate protective levels of the various B vitamins, a good B complex supplement would be a helpful addition to the daily diet.

Antioxidants. Since oxidation reactions and free radical damage may be responsible for some of the changes in the nervous system with aging, an adequate intake of the antioxidant vitamins C, E, and A, and the trace mineral selenium, will provide protection for the nervous system as well as for the body as a whole. It has been proposed, specifically, that vitamin E might retard the production of amyloid, the aluminum-containing substance found in neuritic plaques. Dr. Carl Pfeiffer points out that vitamin E also decreases the oxygen needs of the body's tissues, making more oxygen available for use by the brain's sensitive, oxygen-dependent cells (Pfeiffer 1975, p. 126).

Minerals. Of the mineral nutrients that can help to prevent senile changes in the nervous system, the most important are zinc and magnesium. Zinc is essential to the synthesis of RNA, DNA, and protein, and to the maintenance of vitamin A levels in the blood. Zinc deficiency can cause a confusional state in the elderly, and can produce a decrease in the senses of smell and taste. When older people are not eating properly, zinc deficiency may be at fault, since food is less appetizing when the senses of smell and taste are reduced. (See Table A.4 in the Appendix for a list of zinc-rich foods.)

Magnesium, another important nervous system nutrient, is essential to the transmission of nerve impulses and to muscle contraction, as well as aiding in the absorption of the essential mineral calcium. A list of foods rich in magnesium can be found in Table A.3 in the Appendix.

Choline and lecithin. When students at Northwestern University were given the drug scopolamine, they manifested impairments in memory storage and cognitive functioning that looked like senile behavior, according to Robin Henig in *The Myth of Senility* (1981, p. 180). Scopolamine interferes with the movement of the neurotransmitter acetylcholine in the brain; this brain hormone is crucial to the formation of memory. In animal experiments it has been shown that feeding substances rich in choline, which is required for the synthesis of acetylcholine, resulted in increased amounts of acetylcholine in the hippocampus, the brain's memory center. For this reason, some researchers have recommended an increased dietary intake of choline (available in eggs, fish, and organ meats; see Table A.2 in the Appendix) or lecithin, which contains choline, as a way of promoting proper levels of acetylcholine in the brain.

Drug-nutrient interactions. Besides the danger of consuming too little of essential nutrients, you should be aware that medications that you are taking *may* actually produce nutrient deficiencies. Thus the use of certain medicines may require that added quantities of the nutrients be taken as supplements.

Referring to Table 10.1, find the drug(s) you are presently taking on the left. On the right note which nutrients are depleted by the drug. Simply *add* these nutrients to your diet to counter the negative effects of your prescription drug.

Table 10.1

*Some Commonly Prescribed Drugs
and the Nutrients They Affect*

Drug Trade Name	Major Indication(s) for Use	Major Side Effects	Nutrient(s) Affected
Achromycin	Gram negative and gram positive microorganisms	G.I. systemic irritation Skin rash Kidney: rise in BUN Teeth stained	Reduces absorption of calcium, magnesium, and iron
Aldactazide	Hypertension Congestive heart failure Edema	Drowsiness Lethargy Mental confusion G.I. irritation Menstrual irregularity Headache	Reduced potassium excretion
Aldactone	Hypertension Congestive heart failure Edema	Drowsiness Lethargy Mental confusion G.I. irritation Menstrual irregularity Headache	Reduced potassium excretion
Apresoline	Hypertension	Headache Palpitations	Vitamin B_6 depletion
Aspirin	Minor pain	G.I. irritation	Thiamine and vitamin C deficiency
Atromid-S	Cholesterol control	Nausea Vomiting Loose stools Abdominal distress	Reduction in circulating vitamin K levels

Drug Trade Name	Major Indication(s) for Use	Major Side Effects	Nutrient(s) Affected
Azo Gantanol	Antibacterial Gram negative and gram positive urinary tract infection	Headache Nausea Vomiting Skin rash	Folic acid deficiency
Bentyl with Phenobarbital	Functional G.I. disorders Dizziness	Dry mouth Fatigue	Accelerated vitamin K metabolism
Betapar	Endocrine and rheumatic disorders Collagen and dermatologic disease Hematologic and neoplastic disorders	Fluid retention Muscle weakness G.I. hemorrhage Convulsions	Increased B_6 requirement Increased vitamin C excretion Zinc, potassium deficiency
Brevicon	Oral contraception	Thrombo-phlebitis Pulmonary embolism Cerebral thrombosis Nausea, vomiting Migraine Rash Mental depression	Vitamin B_6 and C depletion
Bronkotabs and Elixir	Bronchial asthma Bronchitis Emphysema	Nervousness Restlessness Sleeplessness	Accelerated vitamin K metabolism

Drug Trade Name	Major Indication(s) for Use	Major Side Effects	Nutrient(s) Affected
Butazolidin	Rheumatoid and osteoarthritis Spondylitis	Edema G.I. distress Rash Confusion Vertigo	Folic acid deficiency
Cantil with Phenobarbital	Lower G.I. distress Diarrhea Abdominal pain Cramping Irritable colon	Dry mouth Blurred vision	Accelerated vitamin K metabolism
Chardonna	Nervous indigestion Gastritis Nausea Vomiting Spastic colon Flatulence	Dry mouth Blurred vision Vertigo Tachycardia	Accelerated vitamin K metabolism
Colbenemid	Chronic gouty arthritis	Headache G.I. distress Urinary frequency Dizziness	Decreased absorption of lactase, fat, sodium, potassium, and B_{12}
Colchicine	Chronic gouty arthritis	Headache G.I. distress Urinary frequency Dizziness	Decreased absorption of lactase, fat, sodium, potassium, and B_{12}
Cortisone tablets and suspension	Adrenocortical deficiency Allergic states Rheumatoid arthritis Dermatoses	Hirsutism and supraclavicular fat pads	Vitamin B_6 deficiency Accelerated vitamin D metabolism Zinc, potassium, and vitamin C deficiency

Drug Trade Name	Major Indication(s) for Use	Major Side Effects	Nutrient(s) Affected
Cortisporin	Burns, wounds Skin grafts Otitis externa Eczema	Systemic intolerance	Reduces lactase levels Vitamin K, B_{12}, and folic acid deficiency
Demulen	Oral contraception	Thrombo-phlebitis Pulmonary embolism Cerebral thrombosis Hemorrhage Myocardial infarction Gallbladder disease	Vitamin B_6 and C depletion
Diethyl-stilbestrol	Menopause Senile vaginitis	Nausea Vomiting Vertigo Anxiety Thirst Rashes	Vitamin B_6 depletion
Diupres	Hypertension	Nausea Vomiting Diarrhea Dizziness Vertigo	Increased magnesium and potassium excretion
Diuril	Hypertension	Nausea Vomiting Diarrhea Dizziness	Increased magnesium and potassium excretion
Doriden	Insomnia	Skin rash	Folic acid deficiency

Drug Trade Name	Major Indication(s) for Use	Major Side Effects	Nutrient(s) Affected
Enovid	Oral contraception	Thrombo-phlebitis Cerebral thrombosis Gallbladder disease	Vitamin B_6 and C depletion
Gantanol	Urinary tract, soft tissue, and respiratory infections	Headache Nausea Vomiting Urticaria Diarrhea Hepatitis	Folic acid deficiency
Hydroten-sion Plus	Hypertension	Headache Palpitations	Vitamin B_6 depletion
Indocin	Rheumatoid arthritis Spondylitis Degenerative joint disease of the hip Gout	G.I. bleeding Headache Dizziness Anorexia Edema Skin rash	Thiamine and vitamin C depletion
Isordil with Phenobarbital	Angina pectoris	Increased intraocular pressure	Accelerated vitamin K metabolism
Lidosporin	Infection pain and itching associated with otitis and furunculosis	Overgrowth of non-susceptible organisms	Malabsorption of vitamins B_{12}, K, and folic acid
Lo-Ovral	Oral contraception	Thrombo-phlebitis Pulmonary embolism Cerebral thrombosis	Vitamin B_6 depletion

Drug Trade Name	Major Indication(s) for Use	Major Side Effects	Nutrient(s) Affected
Mycifradin	Enterocolitis and diarrhea	Nausea Diarrhea	Reduced lactase levels Vitamin K deficiency Malabsorption of vitamin B_{12} and folic acid
Mycolog	Cutaneous candidiasis Infantile eczema	Localized atrophy	Reduced lactase levels Vitamin K deficiency Malabsorption of vitamin B_{12} and folic acid
Neo-Cortef	Contact and allergic dermatitis	Miliaria Folliculitis	Reduced lactase levels Vitamin K deficiency Malabsorption of vitamin B_{12} and folic acid
Neomycin	Suppression of intestinal bacteria Diarrhea	Nausea Vomiting Nephrotoxicity	Reduced lactase levels Vitamin K deficiency Malabsorption of vitamin B_{12} and folic acid
Neosporin	Pseudomonas Staphylococcus bacteria	Overgrowth of non-susceptible organisms	Reduced lactase levels Vitamin K deficiency Malabsorption of vitamin B_{12} and folic acid

Drug Trade Name	Major Indication(s) for Use	Major Side Effects	Nutrient(s) Affected
Norinyl	Oral contraception Hypermenorrhea	Thrombophlebitis Pulmonary embolism Edema G.I. upset	Vitamin B_6 and C depletion
Orasone	Rheumatoid arthritis Joint pain Stiffness Swelling and tenderness	Exaggerated hormonal effects	Increased vitamin B_6 requirement Increased vitamin C excretion Zinc and potassium deficiency
Os-Cal-Mone	Osteoporosis	Uterine bleeding Mastodynia	Vitamin B_6 depletion
Phazyme	G.I. disturbance Aerophagia Dyspepsia Diverticulitis Spastic colitis	None	Accelerated vitamin K metabolism
Polysporin	Gram negative and gram positive microorganisms	Overgrowth of non-susceptible organisms including fungi	Malabsorption of vitamins B_{12}, K, and folic acid
Prednisone	Rheumatoid arthritis Joint pain Stiffness Swelling and tenderness	Exaggerated hormonal effects	Increased vitamin B_{12} requirement Increased vitamin C excretion Zinc and potassium deficiency

Drug Trade Name	Major Indication(s) for Use	Major Side Effects	Nutrient(s) Affected
Premarin	Menopausal syndrome Senile vaginitis Pruritus vulvae	Uterine bleeding Loss of libido	Folic acid deficiency Reduced calcium excretion
Pro-Banthine	Peptic ulcer Hypertrophic gastritis Pancreatitis Diverticulitis Bladder spasm	Dry mouth Blurry vision Urinary retention	Accelerated vitamin K metabolism
Probital	Functional G.I. disorders	Dry mouth Blurry vision Urinary retention	Accelerated vitamin K metabolism
Ser-Ap-Es	Hypertension	Increased gastric secretion Angina-like syndrome Depression Deafness	Vitamin B_6 depletion
Sterazolidin	Anti-arthritic Anti-inflammatory	Edema G.I. upset	Increased vitamin B_6 requirement Increased vitamin C excretion Folic acid, zinc, and potassium deficiency
Sumycin	Gram negative and gram positive microorganisms	G.I. upset Anorexia Nausea Vomiting Diarrhea Dermatitis	Reduced absorption of calcium, magnesium, and iron

Drug Trade Name	Major Indication(s) for Use	Major Side Effects	Nutrient(s) Affected
Tetracyn	Gram negative and gram positive microorganisms	G.I. upset Anorexia Nausea Vomiting Diarrhea Dermatitis	Reduced absorption of calcium, magnesium, and iron

Source: "Index of Nutritional Abnormalities Induced by 50 Commonly Prescribed Drugs," IMA Publications Division, Inter-Marketing Associates, Inc., La Jolla, California, 1978.)

How Environment Influences Mental Functioning

Professor Edwin Boyle of the Miami Heart Institute, has been able to produce improvements in senile symptoms, especially in short-term memory losses, by placing patients in hyperbaric oxygen environments, submarinelike high-pressure chambers with oxygen-rich air. However, the improvements in senile symptoms are only temporary, lasting six weeks to six months after a single treatment (Cheraskin and Ringsdorf 1976, p. 125).

A much more feasible approach in preventing senility may be to maintain a stimulating environment. Even though the process of aging inevitably involves the loss of nerve cells and other physical changes in the nervous system, recent research by Marian Cleeves Diamond at the University of California at Berkeley, suggests that an enriched sensory environment may actually promote the growth of dendrites, at least in animal brains. Dr. Diamond spent fifteen years studying rats raised in three different sorts of environments: "enriched" (twelve rats together in a large cage with mazes, ladders, and tunnels); "deprived" (single rats in small cages); and "standard" (three rats in a similar small cage). On autopsies, the rats' brains showed marked differences:

The rats in the enriched environments, as compared to those in impoverished environments, were found to have a thicker cerebral cortex . . . with more glial cells, increased dendritic branching, less numerous but longer postsynaptic thickening, and an increased RNA/DNA ratio. The studies revealed that cortical changes were different depending on the environments of different age groups over time. . . . Not only have chemical and anatomical studies demonstrated the plasticity of the cortex but they have shown that the net weight of the cortex can increase or decrease at any age studied.

(Diamond 1978)

Diamond believes these findings have implications for old people in nursing homes and other unstimulating environments:

Many early studies on aging human beings were carried out on hospital or mental patients rather than on the normally functioning elderly who have continuously led active lives. It is important to establish which mental alterations are directly determined by the aging machinery and which are due to environment and lack of exercise.

(Diamond 1978)

Diamond's work suggests another key to optimal mental functioning in old age. Besides maintaining good nutrition through wise dietary choices and supplementation of specific nutrients, the best way to ensure continued mental alertness is to maintain an environment that is challenging and stimulating. You *do* have control over the fate of your nervous system!

Nutrients for Other Mental Problems

While senility is the problem that people fear most with advancing age, other problems in mental functioning also trouble older people as they do people of any age. For many of these there are nutritional treatments that may enable you to avoid the dangers of mind-altering drugs and restore proper nutrition to your body's cells at the same time.

We have already mentioned that orthomolecular psychiatry has had pronounced success in treating many schizophrenics with high doses of niacin and other vitamins. Other mental problems may also be related to nutritional deficiencies. As Dr. Richard Kunin observes, there is undoubtedly a connection between the climbing rate of mental illness and the progressive worsening of the American diet. Kunin found that many of his psychiatric patients had marked vitamin and mineral deficiencies, and that their mental status improved with nutritional therapy (Kunin 1980, p. 130).

Insomnia and sleep problems. The need for sleep varies greatly, but the vast majority of the population sleeps between six and nine hours a night. Problems with an inability to fall asleep or stay asleep, early wakening, or lack of refreshing sleep, can lead to serious emotional problems. Sedatives and tranquilizers are widely used—and abused—to induce restful sleep. These drugs can have serious adverse effects in older people, and are better avoided if possible at any age. Perhaps the best natural sleep inducer is a glass of warm milk, which contains the amino ácid tryptophan, a natural tranquilizer which is a precursor of the sedativelike brain hormone serotonin. Present in high concentration in turkey as well as milk, tryptophan should always be taken *in foods*, not as a supplement! Too little is known about the possible deleterious effects of amino acid supplements to take them in megadoses.

Inositol is another natural sleep inducer and anxiety reliever. Contained in lecithin, this B vitamin can be taken in one- to two-gram doses. Calves' brains are a particularly rich source of lecithin.

For people who have difficulty remembering their dreams, the problem may be helped by supplemental vitamin B_6, or pyridoxine. But note that if your dreams wake you up because they are too vivid, you should check your vitamin supplements. If you are taking more than fifty milligrams of vitamin B_6, this may be why you wake up in the midst of colorful dreams. By reducing your intake of this important vitamin your sleep may again become sweet.

Depression. Depression can be a sign of impending nutritional problems. In a classic study of patients with vitamin C deficiencies, Kinsman and Hood found depression to be a universal symptom (Kunin 1980, p. 150). We should view depression as an early warning signal; almost all nutrient and caloric deficiencies produce depression long before they produce physical illness. When you feel depressed, try boosting your vitamin and mineral levels with cautiously increased supplementation.

Anxiety. Anxiety can be expressed in symptoms such as nervousness, fearfulness, or appetite loss. Besides the natural antianxiety foods rich in tryptophan, a vitamin B complex supplement may be helpful. Certain of the B vitamins have specific antianxiety properties, such as inositol and pyridoxine; others are generally useful in protecting against stress, such as niacin and pantothenic acid.

According to Dr. Richard Kunin, high levels of lactic acid in the blood can produce anxiety symptoms. Animals injected with lactic acid were shown to develop anxiety. Because lactic acid binds calcium, depleting calcium stores in the body, it is wise to take supplemental calcium during periods of stress or heavy physical exertion, since both these conditions will produce extra lactic acid. In experimental animals injected with lactate to produce anxiety, calcium injections relieved the anxiety symptoms (Kunin 1980, p. 87). Thus calcium may actually be helpful in relieving anxiety, as well as protecting against depletion of the body's reserves of calcium in the bones and muscles.

Milk is of course a rich source of both calcium *and* tryptophan, which is why we repeat Grandmother's advice: a glass of warm milk before bed!

Rate Your Protective Factors Against Senility

As we have shown, there are definite things that you can do to prevent senility and otherwise keep your brain from deteriorating through time. Now look at the following building block and rate yourself, to see how well you are protecting yourself, or what you need to do to maintain a fit mind.

Building Block #9:

"Keeping Your Marbles:"
Your Protective Factors Against Senility

Maintains a challenging mental life (See p. 166) 10 points	Is aware of physical-mental interactions (See p. 148) 9 points	Eats foods rich in B vitamins (See p. 155) 8 points
Does *not* use tranquilizers or sleeping pills (See pp. 168–169) 7 points	Does not use cocaine or other "recreational" drugs (See p. 167) 6 points	Takes niacin (See p. 154) 5 points
Takes antioxidants (vitamins C, E, A; selenium) (See p. 156) 4 points	Eats zinc-rich foods (See p. 156) 3 points	Eats magnesium-rich foods (See p. 157) 2 points

Total the points for your present protective factors.

Your Score
Block #9 _____

To page 186

⟶

for your next building block

11

RADIANT AGE:

Building Beauty from Within

Looking Healthy Is More Important Than Looking Young!

Age is a great equalizer. No matter how attractive we may have been in our youth, the effects of aging take their toll, turning the glorious golden mane just as gray as the mousy brown, and etching wrinkles across the finely chiseled cheek just as irrevocably as over the plain countenance.

Preoccupation with the outward signs of aging is as old as the history of human civilization. Nearly five thousand years ago the unknown author of the Ebers Papyrus was offering remedies for baldness, wrinkles, and gray hair.

Some rare folks among us, such as Gray Panther leader Maggie Kuhn, make no effort to conceal the signs of age:

> I'm seventy-three years old, and I haven't dyed my hair and I can't afford a face lift. I enjoy my wrinkles and regard them as badges of distinction—I've worked for them!
>
> (Kuhn 1979)

But on the whole, the visible signs of aging generate a degree of anxiety far out of proportion to their seriousness. Vast sums of money are spent on largely useless preparations to prevent or conceal wrinkles and age spots, moisturize dry skin, camouflage gray hair, or "cure" baldness.

Aging, being a great democratic process, presents many people with the opportunity to look relatively better than ever before in their lives. Now, for the first time, the less beautiful have a chance to look as good as their more glamorous peers, simply by taking care to avoid the cosmetic problems that age can bring to us all.

But remember, beauty *is* more than skin-deep, and the truth of this observation becomes increasingly apparent with advancing age. The older we get, the more obvious it becomes that good looks—beyond the accidents of nature that gave us our facial features—are a reflection of good health.

Lin Yutang wisely observed that the objective of older people should not be to look young, but to look *healthy*. For anyone who is no longer able—or willing—to masquerade as a teenager, such a goal is much more realistic, and much more likely to boost one's self-esteem. Many of the unattractive signs of aging are really signs of less than optimal health. As with the justly dreaded killer diseases of middle and old age, the key to a vital, healthy appearance is *prevention*. It's never too early to adopt a sensible routine to forestall the visible, destructive effects of the aging process.

Your Skin: An Outward Mirror of the Aging Process

Function and structure. Wrapped around our bodies at an average thickness of only one twentieth of an inch, our six pounds of skin constitute the largest organ of our body. Within this narrow layer of tissue are contained three vitally important functions. As a protective covering, the skin keeps our body fluids in and harmful materials out. Body temperature is controlled through an intricate network of blood vessels just beneath the skin surface which narrow or dilate to bring varying amounts of blood close to the surface, which is cooled by the evaporation of sweat. Our sense of touch, located in specialized nerve endings in the epidermis (the lining of the skin surface), responds to pain, light touch, deep pressure, warmth, and cold, alerting us to conditions in our environment and affording the complex experience of tactile sensation.

The skin actually consists of four layers. At the bottom, in the basal or growing layer, basal cells divide to produce new cells; these displace the older cells and push them upward through a "clear cell" layer and a granular layer, until they finally reach the outer, keratinized layer. The whole process takes three to four weeks in humans. The cells produce granular material as they mature; this material eventually causes the cells to consolidate into a thick, tough material in the outer keratin layer. The cells eventually slough off from this protective outer layer of skin, carrying away large molecules of waste material with them (Jones 1976).

The aging process in the skin. While the skin continues to perform its functions at about the same efficiency throughout life, its appearance can be markedly affected by the aging process. One of the most noticeable changes results from alterations in the collagen, the protein substance which gives the skin its elasticity.

You have undoubtedly noticed that a baby's skin is very soft and jellylike. As the skin matures, chemical bridges known as cross-linkages, form between the collagen molecules, binding them together into larger, more unwieldy molecules. Collagen molecules must be cross-linked to some extent in order for the skin to be supple and elastic. However, as we get older, the normal cross-linkage processes in our collagen tissues begin to outstrip the enzymatic repair mechanisms that normally reverse cross-linkages and maintain a balance in the process. As cross-linkages proliferate, the skin loses its elasticity and becomes hard and leathery.

Cross-linkage has been attributed to the action of free radicals, those highly reactive portions of molecules that will combine with anything in their path once they are set loose in the body. Among the sources of free radicals are the ultraviolet rays in sunlight, cigarette smoke, and oxidative processes, some of which arise from the foods we eat. We will soon see how some inexpensive nutrients, known as antioxidants, act to destroy these harmful free radicals. Other sources of damage to the skin include heat, wind, and harsh chemicals as in soaps.

As the skin ages—thinning from the loss of subcutaneous tissues and epidermis, and getting more leathery from cross-linkage—wrinkles become increasingly pronounced. Some people elect to have facelift operations, which can cost in the thousands of dollars. Other surgical approaches to wrinkling include peeling away the superficial layers of the skin through the use of chemicals, and dermabrasion, or "sandpaper surgery." Some people have even resorted to the use of hemorrhoid ointment as a means of temporarily tightening the skin around the eyes!

Other problems of the aging skin inspire less drastic measures, though they can be equally disturbing. The skin as it ages becomes dry and flaky, owing to a decrease in the activity of the oil and sweat glands and a consequent loss of its natural moisturizing ability. This dryness and its frequent accompaniment, itching, can become especially troublesome during the winter months when indoor heating tends to dry out the air and aggravate the condition.

Recently information has appeared in popular health magazines concerning collagen as a new "miracle cure" for the wrinkling and dryness of aging skin. This information is largely undocumented, supplied by the European exporter of the original collagen products. It is unlikely that putting collagen on the outside of your skin is going to make any difference in what is going on *inside*—and since the skin is continually regenerating itself, that's where to attack the problem. As you will see in this chapter, a few key nutrients will help your body manufacture healthy collagen. For these reasons, we do *not* recommend that you spend your precious dollars to purchase these would-be miracle skin creams.

In Mediterranean countries, olive oil has been rubbed on the skin to lubricate it and prevent the loss of moisture since antiquity—a much less expensive cosmetic approach, and one with a much longer history of satisfied users. We heartily continue to recommend this "treatment" for skin of any age.

Another cosmetically disturbing problem for many older people is the appearance of "liver spots" or "age spots," areas of brownish pigmentation that tend to accumulate especially on the back of the hands, the forehead, and cheeks. These age spots consist of the pigment lipofuscin. It is not known whether lipofuscin is harmful or not, but besides the skin, it has been noted to accumulate in the brain and other nerve cells, and in heart and other muscle cells, with advancing age. This age pigment is believed to be a by-product of lipid peroxidation, a free-radical reaction of fats in the cells similar to the process of oils becoming rancid. Cosmetic bleaching creams, usually containing ammoniated mercury or hydroquinone, are widely advertised to cope with this problem (Lubowe 1976). While these creams may act locally to reduce melanocyte production, they of course do nothing to halt the underlying processes of aging. Certainly it is not desirable to use *any* cosmetic that contains compounds of the highly toxic metal mercury.

A diet for healthy skin. We cannot pretend that nutrition is the *only* key to maintaining healthy, moist, unlined skin. Environmental factors are also extremely important, as we will show later. But poor nutrition is certainly one of the main causes of premature aging of the skin. As is the case with any organ that is constantly repairing and replenishing itself through the creation of new cells, the quality of the skin depends on the quality of the raw materials from which its cells are constructed. Our skin is a direct reflection of our diet.

The nutritional foundation for healthy, smooth skin is the same preventive diet that we have been advocating throughout this book. Such a diet eliminates refined carbohydrates and junk food, and avoids caffeine which can exhaust the endocrine system. It is low in fats and supplies adequate protein through a combination of vegetable sources (whole grains, seeds, and legumes), dairy, eggs, and the sparing use of fish, poultry, and perhaps small quantities of *lean* red meats. Plenty of fresh fruits and vegetables are essential, not only for the nutrients they supply, but also for the maintenance of proper acid-alkali balance.

Remember also that it is unwise to use *excessive* quantities of polyunsaturated fats in the diet, which can be a source of damaging free radicals—one of the underlying causes of skin wrinkling.

Because our caloric requirements decrease with age, this preventive diet will probably need to be supplemented with vitamins and minerals to ensure adequate levels of nutrients vital to skin health.

Vitamin A is essential to the formation of healthy cells in the basal layer of the skin, which eventually move out to the surface. This vitamin also helps to promote the skin's natural moisture. *Vitamin D* is helpful in treating dry skin. Both these vitamins may be especially deficient during the winter—vitamin D because of the reduced amount of sunlight, and vitamin A because it may not be supplied as adequately by dairy products during the months when cows are not grazing on fresh grass. Thus, during the winter months, when dry skin can be a particular problem, it may be beneficial to provide these vitamins by supplementing the diet with halibut or cod liver oil or fresh wheat germ oil.

One of the symptoms of scurvy, the *vitamin C* deficiency disease, is poor skin condition. While Americans are in little danger of developing full-blown scurvy these days, it is likely that relatively high doses of this antioxidant vitamin can help to slow down the aging process in general, including a retardation of skin wrinkling. Vitamin C is also essential to the formation of collagen—the protein substance that makes up skin and other connective tissue.

Adelle Davis reported that a deficiency of vitamin B_2, or riboflavin, at *any* age, may be characterized by peculiar vertical wrinkles around the mouth which she called whistle marks. This condition is particularly prevalent among aging women because of their thinner skin (Davis 1970, p. 91). A good vitamin B complex supplement will provide riboflavin to protect against this problem, as well as other necessary B vitamins.

In the 1970s Dr. Benjamin Frank popularized a "No-Aging Diet" consisting of foods that were high in nucleic acids (RNA and DNA), such as seafoods and yeast. Among the benefits claimed for this diet was the disappearance of wrinkles and facial lines, the fading of age spots, and the restoration of moisture and a healthy glow to the skin. This may all sound too good to be true, and sure enough, there was a general rush among medical experts to debunk Frank's claims. Among other criticisms, detractors questioned whether the consumption of large quantities of nucleic-acid-rich foods would result in high levels of nucleic acids in the cells, where they were needed. Secondly, it was pointed out that such a diet could be dangerous for anyone with a tendency toward gout, since the high-nucleic-acid diet produces high levels of uric acid in the blood.

Very recently, a paper by Ames and co-workers at the University of California at Berkeley, and the University of Southern California (Ames et al. 1981), hypothesizes that high plasma uric acid may be a *protective* mechanism developed through human evolution, and may act as one of the most potent antioxidants in the human body. If this proves to be the case, then the nucleic-acid diet may be due for closer scrutiny. While we cannot at this point advocate a high-nucleic-acid diet for everyone, you might try shifting your diet toward somewhat increased quantities of seafood including shellfish, sardines, herring, and anchovies, and such fresh fish as halibut, bass, salmon, tuna, trout, flounder, and scrod; liver and other organ meats such as kidneys; and yeast, spinach, oatmeal, and other nucleic-acid-rich "superfoods." Remember to exercise caution, however; for one thing, as anyone who has eaten an anchovy can readily testify, some of these foods are extremely high in salt content, and excessive sodium intake is to be discouraged. A high-fluid intake is also advised.

Minerals that promote skin health include *calcium* and *magnesium* (which can be supplied in a balanced supplement such as dolomite), *zinc, manganese,* and *potassium*.

Topical applications of nutrients. Some of the nutrients recommended as dietary supplements are also beneficial when applied externally. Vitamin E oil and vitamins A and D ointment are among the best treatments for dry skin.

Dr. Albert Kligman, founder of a clinic for aging skin at the University of Pennsylvania Medical School, has been using a special preparation known as vitamin A acid experimentally, to smooth out skin that is showing only early signs of wrinkling. Originally developed as a treatment for acne, the vitamin A acid is available only by prescription and has not yet been officially approved for aging skin (Padus 1981).

It is significant that the best-known protection against one of the greatest sources of damage to the skin, namely excessive exposure to sunlight, is also a nutrient—the B vitamin para-aminobenzoic acid, or PABA. This vitamin is used in many commercially available sunscreen lotions and creams. In a study comparing twenty-four commercial sunscreen preparations, PABA was shown to be the most effective (Pathak et al. 1968). This beneficial vitamin blocks out the harmful portions of the ultraviolet spectrum while allowing the less dangerous, tanning rays of the sun to come through.

Avoid excess sun; quit smoking. We can't stress strongly enough the importance of avoiding excess exposure to the sun if you want to prevent premature aging of the skin. People with light complexions and blue or green eyes are the most susceptible to sun damage; those with black skin are most resistant. Incidentally, in general, black skin is less subject to the effects of aging.

Sun damage is cumulative, and so the proper prevention of wrinkles begins early in life. We repeat, please limit your exposure to sunlight, and always use a sunscreen preparation (preferably one containing PABA) when you are outdoors. Not only will these precautions prevent UV damage and wrinkles, but they can also prevent sun-induced cancer.

Another often overlooked cause of skin wrinkling is cigarette smoking. This connection was brought home dramatically by Dr. Harry Daniell of California, who assigned a "wrinkle score" to each of 1,104 subjects, aged 30–70, based on the severity of wrinkling in the "crow's foot" area at the corner of the eye. He found that in each age group the most heavily wrinkled people were the smokers. For example, smokers in the 40–49-year age group were as likely to be prominently wrinkled as nonsmokers twenty years their senior! In his study, Dr. Daniell found that wrinkling was even more strongly associated with smoking than it was with outdoor exposure (Daniell 1971). While this was only one study, and while the methodology might not have met strict laboratory standards, Dr. Daniell's conclusions should certainly give smokers yet one more reason to consider giving up their harmful habit.

It's unfortunate that such pleasurable activities as sunning are so damaging to our skin. Another culprit is bathing—especially those soothing, hot baths so many of us like to submerge ourselves in. Excessive bathing, especially in hot water, can aggravate skin dryness and may lead to itching. If you have these skin problems, take warm showers rather than soaking in a hot tub, avoid harsh soaps, and use an after-bath skin oil. While there are many "itch remedies" available at your local pharmacy, remember that some of these can produce irritations and allergic reactions in sensitive individuals. The best and safest skin treatment we have found for itching and other allergic reactions is colloidal oatmeal. It is available in any pharmacy without a prescription.

Remember also that your clothing may aggravate itching. Avoid synthetic fabrics and try wearing 100-percent cotton, also avoiding fabric softeners and other chemicals that can come in contact with your skin.

Nourishing Your Hair

Manufactured within the hair follicles in the skin, the hairs on your head number somewhere in the neighborhood of 120,000, and grow at a rate of $\frac{1}{16}$ to $\frac{1}{8}$ of an inch a day, or five inches a year. The hair is composed of 90-percent protein, and it has been shown that when extra protein was provided in the diet in the form of 14 grams of gelatin daily, the individual hair strands increased in diameter (Kolodzey 1981).

Hair loss. As with the skin, the hair undergoes characteristic changes with aging. Scalp hair becomes increasingly thin and lifeless, while hair growth may increase on the cheeks, chin, and lips. Women, as well as men, may experience balding, though the pattern of hair loss tends to be more diffuse in women. The perspiration and oil glands in the scalp also tend to work less efficiently with age.

The ancient Egyptians were apparently as worried about balding as we are today—if we can take their remedies as any indication. The Ebers Papyrus suggests that the "Bald One" rub on his head a concoction of "Fat-of-the-Lion, Fat-of-the-Hippopotamus, Fat-of-the-Crocodile, Fat-of-the-Cat, Fat-of-the-Serpent, and Fat-of-the-Egyptian Goat." Another balding remedy is even more revolting: "Writing-fluid, Fat-of-the-Hippopotamus, and Gazelle's Dung."

Whether these preparations ever succeeded in restoring hair growth is questionable; but the search for potions to preserve or restore hair continues today. While we cannot offer any nutritional panaceas for this universally dreaded sign of aging, we can suggest some possible nutritional causes of *excessive* hair loss that is not purely a manifestation of genetic balding patterns.

Excess copper in the blood can produce hair loss. Both birth control pills and third-trimester pregnancy are associated with elevated levels of serum copper. Women taking birth control pills should discontinue them immediately if excessive hair loss occurs. Drinking water may also contain high concentrations of copper.

Selenium can also cause hair loss. Beware of over supplementation with this highly toxic trace mineral. See chapter 2 for a full discussion of this important antioxidant.

Among the nutrient deficiencies which may be connected with excessive hair loss are vitamin B_6, zinc, and sulfur. Stress, so common in our modern life-style, can contribute to hair loss and appears to be an increasing problem in female baldness as more and more women are exposed to the stresses of modern business and industry. To protect against stress your best insurance is supplementation of vitamin B complex, as well as adequate protein

and vitamin E. Egg yolks are a good source of the helpful
B vitamin biotin as well as sulfur. Folic acid deficiency can
also lead to hair loss; men with baldness may well have
high individual requirements for this and other B vitamins
which are not being met by their diet.

Graying. One of the commonest accompaniments of
aging is graying of the hair. It may be that, besides hereditary factors, nutrition may play a role. Graying may also
be a manifestation of more generalized aging processes. In
a study performed in Mexico between 1948 and 1969, it
was found that of the 480 Mexicans studied, in each age
category those with gray hair at the beginning of the study
had a higher mortality rate than those whose hair hadn't
turned gray (Lasker and Kaplan 1975).

If graying of the hair is in fact an indicator of the rate
of aging, then one possible antigraying approach would be
to use high doses of the antiaging nutrients as dietary
supplements. Dr. Abram Hoffer reports that when his hair
began to turn gray over ten years ago he started taking 800
IU of vitamin E daily. To his surprise his hair color was
restored (Hoffer and Walker 1980, p. 126)!

Back in the 1940s it was first reported that high doses
of the B vitamin PABA produced a darkening of gray hair.
In one study, Dr. B. F. Sieve found some restoration of
hair color in 70 percent of subjects given 200 milligrams of
PABA a day (Sieve 1941). Zarafonetis (1960) reported darkening of gray hair as an incidental finding in some patients
receiving very high doses of PABA for unrelated medical
problems.

It has also been suggested that zinc may help with
graying hair, while others have made claims for pantothenic acid, a B vitamin. An "antigraying formula" consisting of 300 milligrams each of pantothenic acid and PABA,
as well as 5 milligrams of folic acid and other B vitamins in
adequate quantities, has been reported to return gray hair
to its original color in some cases (Mann 1980, p. 71).

We certainly can't promise that any of these supplements will help in any given case to reverse hair graying.
If you are taking nutritional supplements as a general
safeguard against the aging process, it is of course possible
that you *may* experience the unexpected additional benefit

of restored hair color. Such claims have also been made for nucleic-acid-rich diets. If so, then the explanation most likely lies in improved overall nutritional status and slowed rate of aging, rather than any magical effect of a single nutrient on hair color per se.

You Don't Need to Lose Your Teeth

Even if your hair turns gray and your skin becomes wrinkled, you most definitely do *not* have to lose your teeth as an inevitable part of the aging process. Tooth loss becomes an increasing threat with advancing age because of the increased incidence of periodontal disease, that inflammation of the gums caused by bacterial accumulations on the teeth that leads to loss of the supporting bone structure. According to the National Health Survey from 1960 to 1962, by 60 years of age, 35 percent of the American public had lost *all* their teeth (Cheraskin et al. 1968)! Periodontal disease, which has been observed in 70 percent or more of subjects over the age of 45 in one study, is the single greatest cause of loss of teeth in adults (Peterson 1972).

Dental problems begin in childhood with carious disease. As reported by Cheraskin and his co-workers, dental caries is strongly associated in its geographic distribution with the occurrence of such other "diseases of civilization" as coronary artery disease, obesity, diabetes, elevated triglycerides, and cancer of the digestive tract. A common underlying factor in all these conditions is the modern "civilized" diet, which is high in refined carbohydrates which are known to be a causative factor in dental caries (Cheraskin et al. 1968, p. 315). The *Streptococcus mutans* bacteria that produce dental caries, thrive on sugar, using it not only for energy, but also as a component of the plaque they deposit on the teeth. These bacteria also produce lactic acid which eats away at the teeth. Plaque, as we have all heard so often, is also the starting point for periodontal disease, and this is why it's so important to maintain a regular program of dental hygiene to remove the daily buildup of this substance which threatens to rob us of our teeth, as the serious threat of periodontal disease increases with increasing age.

Besides avoiding simple sugars and other refined carbohydrates, you should avoid excessive meat, which is a source of phosphorus which can leach the calcium out of the bones. Similarly, *any* soft drinks, not just those containing sugar, are to be avoided, since they too contain large amounts of phosphorus in the form of phosphoric acid (Fellman 1981).

Too much phosphorus and not enough calcium is a major factor in the periodontal bone loss that causes so many Americans to lose their teeth. Reduced protein consumption and a calcium-magnesium supplement such as dolomite, supplying about 1,000 milligrams of calcium daily, will provide protection.

Vitamin C deficiency, or scurvy, is characterized by gum disease among other symptoms. It has recently been shown experimentally that "subclinical vitamin-C deficiency significantly increases susceptibility to periodontal disease (Alvares 1981).

Some foods appear to be beneficial in fighting dental caries, plaque, and periodontal disease. Green leafy vegetables, eaten raw in the form of salads, are a good daily form of dental insurance. Cheese reportedly reduces the amount of acid produced by bacteria, and carrots and bananas make bacteria clump together, facilitating their removal through brushing and flossing. The citric acid in citrus fruits loosens plaque, making it easier to remove. As reported in *Prevention* magazine, Professor Kenneth O. Madsen has also found that seed coverings, such as sunflower and oat hulls, rice, corn and oat bran, whole wheat, and other seed hulls, appear for unknown reasons to decrease dental caries as much as 78 percent when incorporated into the diets of laboratory rodents. He therefore suggests that these healthful fibrous substances, so often removed from our diet, be incorporated into snack foods to provide protection for our teeth (Fellman 1981).

Nails

If you are troubled with brittle, cracking nails or even lose them, zinc may be the answer to this nutritional riddle. We have helped numerous women with these problems and, without exception, 30 milligrams of zinc every day restored flexibility and health to the "windows of the hands." If you prefer, you can eat foods rich in zinc, including brewer's yeast, oysters, shellfish, liver, soybeans, spinach, and sunflower seeds. In addition to encouraging nail strength you may additionally benefit by experiencing quicker wound healing, reduced cholesterol deposits, a better appetite, a restoration of taste, and less fatigue—all related, in some cases, to a deficiency in nature's healing mineral, zinc.

Rate Your Protective Factors for Healthy Good Looks

By following these tips your skin, teeth, nails, and hair, will last as long as you do! Now look at the following building block, and you'll see that beauty is more than skin-deep.

Building Block #10:

"Keeping Your Looks:"
Your Protective Factors for Healthy Good Looks

Takes vitamin A, E, & C supplements (See p. 177) **10 points**	Avoids strong sunlight without sunscreen (See p. 179) **9 points**	Avoids tobacco & rooms with tobacco smoke (See p. 179) **8 points**
Avoids high-fat, high-refined-carbohydrate diet (See p. 176) **7 points**	Eats carrots, bananas, & citrus fruits to protect teeth (See p. 184) **6 points**	Eats nucleic-acid-rich foods* (See p. 179) **5 points**
Takes zinc for strong nails (See p. 185) **4 points**	Takes B complex vitamins for hair (See p. 181) **3 points**	Coats skin regularly with olive oil (See p. 175) **2 points**

Total the points for your present   Your Score
protective factors.   Block #10 _____

* CAUTION: These foods are contraindicated for the gout-prone individual.

To page 187

for your "Pyramid of Healthful Aging"

The Pyramid of Healthful Aging

Insert your scores from the building blocks on ·the pages indicated. All of your totals. Then, to see where you fit in the optimal scheme, see the scale that follows.

At three-month intervals we strongly recommend that you again score yourself. In this way you work toward living, loving, and looking well for the rest of your life!

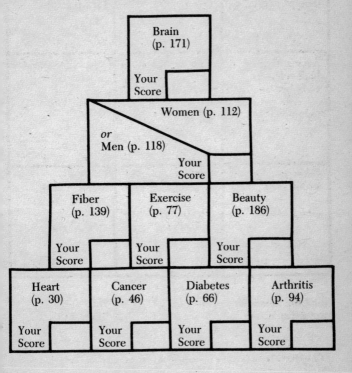

Brain
(p. 171)

Your Score

Women (p. 112)

or
Men (p. 118)

Your Score

Fiber
(p. 139)

Your Score

Exercise
(p. 77)

Your Score

Beauty
(p. 186)

Your Score

Heart
(p. 30)

Your Score

Cancer
(p. 46)

Your Score

Diabetes
(p. 66)

Your Score

Arthritis
(p. 94)

Your Score

To page 188

for rating scale

Your Protective Health Rating

Scores Between	Rating
450 – 486	A+
400 – 449	A
350 – 399	B+
300 – 349	B
250 – 299	B–
200 – 249	Average
150 – 199	D
below 150	F

12

DOING IT DAY TO DAY

As you can see, the dietary adjustments I call for throughout this book are relatively easy to achieve. Most of the foods are already part of your regular diet. The vitamins and minerals are readily available and have been kept to a minimum amount.

There are no "secrets," never before discovered as in so many diet and health books. The dietary changes are highly individualistic and can be achieved with most ethnic cuisines or even by shifting proportions with average American foods. The end result, in all cases, is a well-balanced diet plan that yields healthful aging, longer life, and an increased vigor.

A Note about Dosages

The best way to receive the nutrients you need for a long life is *primarily* through the foods you eat and the liquids you drink. Just taking extra supplements does not assure you that increased levels of these nutrients will appear in your blood. Our body, through its own methods of governance, controls the levels of most nutrients in our bloodstream and may excrete excess quantities of various nutrients.

Nevertheless, most of us need the extra nutrients suggested in the building blocks, but only in conjunction with the foods suggested. Supplements, though they are great in compensating for our devitalized soils and foods, and lifetimes of faulty eating, are not a substitute for wise diets.

Having said all this I would like to emphasize that within the constraints of being unable to suggest with precise accuracy your particular dosage requirements for the various nutrients discussed throughout the book, I have tried to suggest the *ranges* of supplementation generally recommended by practitioners. To more accurately determine how much you may need to take of each vitamin and mineral complex laboratory analyses must be undertaken and your reactions to various dosages watched. For this reason the *supplement ranges* (SRs) listed in Tables 1 and 2 in addition to the ranges listed in the building blocks and within each chapter, should enable you to begin your program without any difficulty.

By and large, most readers will be like my typical patient and do well to take a high potency, multivitamin/mineral supplement as a basic formula. Be certain this formula contains at least 200 IUs of Vitamin E, 50 mcg. of biotin (the two most expensive nutrients to package and good indicators of the quality of the formulation), 50 mg. of each of the B vitamins, 30 mg. of zinc, selenium (at *least* 10 mcg., no more than 100 mcg.), and chromium (at least 15 mcg.) In addition to these nutrients your basic formula will, of course contain the usual amounts of vitamins A and D and a good range of minerals. I do not recommend specific brands, but several excellent formulas are readily available in most quality health food stores. Be sure the one you pick contains the nutrients in the quantities suggested.

In addition to this basic formulation you will want to take the specific vitamins and minerals called for in each building block to achieve your desired scores and then the highest grade in the pyramid of healthful aging. You will have a good idea of how much to add of each nutrient depending upon how you score in each building block when you first read this book, and also according to your predisposition to the diseases discussed. For more specific knowledge of your nutrient levels you will need blood and hair assays.

The following tables give the supplement ranges for the vitamins and minerals discussed throughout this book. In addition I list food sources, the body parts affected (by the nutrient), bodily functions facilitated, deficiency symptoms, and therapeutic indications. As in all such general aids these tables are *not* intended for diagnostic or prescriptive purposes; for any illness please see your physician and use these charts during your discussion about appropriate therapy.

Table 1

Vitamins and Their Uses*

Vitamin	Source	Body Parts Affected	Bodily Functions Facilitated	Deficiency Symptoms	Therapeutic Indications
A Fat Soluble Augmenting Nutrients: B complex, choline, C, D, E, calcium, phosphorus, zinc SR = 20,000–100,000 IU	green & yellow fruits & vegetables, milk, milk products, fish liver oil apricots (dried): 1 cup = 16,000 IU liver (beef): ¼ lb. = 50,000 IU spinach (cooked): 1 cup = 8,000 IU carrots (raw) 1 med. = 10,000 IU	bones, eyes, skin, soft tissue, teeth	body tissue reparation & maintenance (resist infection), visual purple production (necessary for night vision)	allergies, appetite loss, blemishes, dry hair, fatigue, itching, burning eyes, loss of smell, night blindness, rough dry skin, sinus trouble, soft tooth enamel, susceptibility to infections	acne, alcoholism, allergies, arthritis, asthma, athlete's foot, bronchitis, colds, cystitis, diabetes, eczema, heart disease, hepatitis, migraine headaches, psoriasis, sinusitis, stress, tooth & gum disorders

192

| B Water Soluble Augmenting Nutrients: C, E, calcium, phosphorus SR = see each | brewer's yeast, whole liver, grains | eyes, gastro-intestinal tract, hair, liver, mouth, nerves, skin | energy, metabolism (carbohydrate, fat, protein), muscle tone maintenance (gastrointestinal tract) | acne, anemia, constipation, cholesterol (high), digestive disturbances, fatigue, hair (dull, dry, falling), insomnia, skin (dry, rough) | alcoholic psychosis, allergies, anemia, baldness, barbiturate overdose, cystitis, heart abnormalities, hypoglycemia, hypersensitive children, Menière's syndrome, menstrual difficulties, migraine headaches, overweight, postoperative nausea, stress |

Vitamin	Source	Body Parts Affected	Bodily Functions Facilitated	Deficiency Symptoms	Therapeutic Indications
B$_1$ Thiamin Water Soluble Augmenting Nutrients: B complex, B$_2$, folic acid, niacin, C, E, manganese, sulfur SR = 50 mg.- several grams	blackstrap molasses, brewer's yeast, brown rice, fish, meat, nuts, organ meats, poultry, wheat germ brewer's yeast: 2 tbsp. = 3 mg. peanuts: 1¼ cups = 1 mg. sunflower seeds: 1 cup = 2 mg. Brazil nuts: 1 cup = 3 mg.	brain, ears, eyes, hair, heart, nervous system	appetite, blood building, carbohydrate metabolism, digestion (hydrochloric acid production), energy, growth, learning capacity, muscle tone maintenance (intestines, stomach, heart)	appetite loss, digestive disturbances, fatigue, irritability, nervousness, numbness of hands & feet, pain & noise sensitivity, pains around heart, shortness of breath	alcoholism, anemia, congestive heart failure, constipation, diarrhea, diabetes, indigestion, nausea, mental illness, pain (alleviates), rapid heart rate, stress
B$_2$ Riboflavin Water Soluble Augmenting Nutrients:	blackstrap molasses, nuts, organ meats, whole grains almonds:	eyes, hair, nails, skin, soft body tissue	antibody & red blood cell formation, cell respiration, metabolism	cataracts, corner of mouth cracks & sores, dizziness, itching burning eyes, poor	acne, alcoholism, arthritis, athlete's foot, baldness, cataracts, diabetes, diarrhea,

194

B complex, B6, niacin, C, phosphorus SR = 50 mg.-several grams	1 cup = 1 mg. brussels sprouts: 1 cup = 2 mg. brewer's yeast: 3 tbsp. = 1 mg. liver (beef): ¼ lb. = 5 mg.		(carbohydrate, fat, protein)	digestion, retarded growth, red sore tongue	indigestion, stress
B6 Pyridoxine Water Soluble Augmenting Nutrients: B complex, B1, B2, pantothenic acid, C, magnesium, potassium, linoleic acid, sodium SR = 50 mg.-several grams	blackstrap molasses, brewer's yeast, green leafy vegetables, meat, organ meats, wheat germ, whole grains, desiccated liver liver (beef): ¼ lb. = 1 mg. prunes (cooked): 1 cup = 2 mg. brown rice: 1 cup = 2 mg. peas: 1 cup = 2 mg.	blood, muscles, nerves, skin	antibody formation, digestion (hydrochloric acid production), fat & protein utilization (weight control), maintains sodium/potassium balance (nerves)	acne, anemia, arthritis, convulsions in babies, depression, dizziness, hair loss, irritability, learning disabilities, weakness	atherosclerosis, baldness, cholesterol (high), cystitis, facial oiliness, hypoglycemia, mental retardation, muscular disorders, nervous disorders, nausea in pregnancy, overweight, postoperative nausea, stress, sun sensitivity

195

Vitamin	Source	Body Parts Affected	Bodily Functions Facilitated	Deficiency Symptoms	Therapeutic Indications
B_{12} Cobalamin Water Soluble Augmenting Nutrients: B complex, B_6, choline, inositol, C, potassium, sodium SR = 50–100 mcg.	cheese, fish, milk, milk products, organ meats, cottage cheese liver (beef): ¼ lb. = 90 mcg. tuna fish (canned): ½ lb. = 5 mcg. eggs: 1 med. = 1 mcg. milk: 1 cup = 1 mcg.	blood, nerves	appetite, blood cell formation, cell longevity, health nervous system, metabolism (carbohydrate, fat, protein)	general weakness, nervousness, pernicious anemia, walking & speaking difficulties	alcoholism, allergies, anemia, arthritis, bronchial asthma, bursitis, epilepsy, fatigue, hypoglycemia, insomnia, overweight, shingles, stress
Biotin B Complex Water Soluble Augmenting Nutrients: B complex, B_{12}, folic acid,	legumes, whole grains, organ meats brewer's yeast: 1 tbsp. = 20 mcg. lentils: 1 cup = 25 mcg.	hair, muscles, skin	cell growth, fatty acid production, metabolism (carbohydrate, fat, protein), vitamin B utilization	depression, dry skin, fatigue, grayish skin color, insomnia, muscular pain, poor appetite	baldness, dermatitis, eczema, leg cramps

196

Nutrient	Food Sources	Body Parts	Body Functions	Deficiency Symptoms	Overdose
pantothenic acid, C, sulfur SR = 50–500 mcg.	mung bean sprouts: 1 cup = 200 mcg. egg yolk: 1 med. = 10 mcg. liver (beef): ¼ lb. = 112 mcg. soybeans: 1 cup = 120 mcg.				
Choline B Complex Water Soluble Augmenting Nutrients: A, B complex, B₁₂, folic acid, inositol, linoleic acid SR = 500 mg.- several grams	brewer's yeast, fish, legumes, organ meats, soybeans, wheat germ, lecithin liver (beef): ¼ lb. = 500 mg. egg yolks: 1 med. = 250 mg. peanuts (roasted with skin): ½ cup = 190 mg.	hair, kidneys, liver, thymus gland	lecithin formation, liver & gallbladder regulation, metabolism (fats, cholesterol), nerve transmission	bleeding stomach ulcers, growth problems, heart trouble, high blood pressure, impaired liver & kidney function, intolerance to fats	alcoholism, atherosclerosis, baldness, cholesterol (high), constipation, dizziness, ear noises, hardening of the arteries, headaches, heart trouble, high blood pressure, hypoglycemia, insomnia

Vitamin	Source	Body Parts Affected	Bodily Functions Facilitated	Deficiency Symptoms	Therapeutic Indications
Folic Acid Folacin B Complex Water Soluble Augmenting Nutrients: B complex, B₁₂, biotin, pantothenic acid, C SR = 400 mcg.- low mg. level	green leafy vegetables, milk, milk products, organ meats, oysters, salmon, whole grains brewer's yeast: 1 tbsp. = 200 mcg. dates (dried): 1 med. = 2,500 mcg. spinach (steamed): 1 cup = 448 mcg. tuna fish (canned): ¼ lb. = 2,250 mcg.	blood, glands, liver	appetite, body growth & reproduction, hydrochloric acid production, protein metabolism, red blood cell formation	anemia, digestive disturbances, graying hair, growth problems	alcoholism, anemia, atherosclerosis, baldness, diarrhea, fatigue, menstrual problems, mental illness, stomach ulcers, stress
Inositol B Complex Water Soluble	blackstrap molasses, citrus fruits, brewer's	brain, hair, heart, kidneys,	artery hardening retardation, cholesterol	cholesterol (high), constipation, eczema, eye	atherosclerosis, baldness, cholesterol (high),

198

Nutrient	Food Sources	Body Part	Function	Deficiency Symptoms	Ailments
Augmenting Nutrients: B complex, B_{12}, choline, linoleic acid SR = 500 mg.- several grams	yeast, meat, milk, nuts, vegetables, whole grains, lecithin oranges (fresh): 1 med. = 400 mg. grapefruit: 1 med. = 500 mg. peanuts (roasted with skin): 1 cup = 400 mg.	liver, muscles	reduction, hair growth, lecithin formation, metabolism (fat & cholesterol)	abnormalities, hair loss	constipation, heart disease, overweight
Niacin Niacinamide B Complex Water Soluble Augmenting Nutrients: B complex, B_1, B_2, C, Phosphorus SR = 250 mg.- several grams	brewer's yeast, lean meats, milk products, poultry, desiccated liver rhubarb (cooked): 1 cup = 80 mg. chicken breast (fried): ½ lb. = 25 mg. peanuts (roasted with skin): 1 cup = 40 mg.	brain, liver, nerves, skin, soft tissue, tongue	circulation, cholesterol level reduction, growth, hydrochloric acid production, metabolism (protein, fat) sex hormone production	appetite loss, canker sores, depression, fatigue, halitosis, headaches, indigestion, insomnia, muscular weakness, nausea, nervous disorders, skin eruptions	acne, baldness, diarrhea, halitosis, high blood pressure, leg cramps, migraine headaches, poor circulation, stress, tooth decay

Vitamin	Source	Body Parts Affected	Bodily Functions Facilitated	Deficiency Symptoms	Therapeutic Indications
Pantothenic Acid B Complex Water Soluble Augmenting Nutrients: B complex, B₆, B₁₂, biotin, folic acid, C SR = 50 mg.- several grams	brewer's yeast, legumes, organ meats, salmon, wheat germ, whole grains liver (beef): ¼ lb. = 8 mg. mushrooms (cooked): 1 cup = 82 mg. elderberries (raw): 1 cup = 45 mg.	adrenal glands, digestive tract, nerves, skin	antibody formation, carbohydrate, fat, protein conversion (energy), growth stimulation, vitamin utilization	diarrhea, duodenal ulcers, eczema, hypoglycemia, intestinal disorders, kidney trouble, loss of hair, muscle cramps, premature aging, respiratory infections, restlessness, nerve problems, sore feet, vomiting	allergies, arthritis, baldness, cystitis, digestive disorders, hypoglycemia, tooth decay, stress
PABA Para Aminobenzoic Acid Water Soluble Augmenting Nutrients: B complex, folic acid, C SR = 50–500 mg.	blackstrap molasses, brewer's yeast, liver, organ meats, wheat germ	glands, hair, intestines, skin	blood cell formation, graying hair (color restoration), intestinal bacteria activity, protein metabolism	constipation, depression, digestive disorders, fatigue, gray hair, headaches, irritability	baldness, graying hair, overactive thyroid gland, parasitic diseases, rheumatic fever, stress, infertility. External: burns, dark skin spots, dry skin, sunburn, wrinkles

200

	Food Sources	Body Parts	Functions	Deficiency Symptoms	Therapeutic Uses
B15 Pangamic Acid Water Soluble Augmenting Nutrients: B complex, C, E SR = no longer available	brewer's yeast, brown rice, meat (rare), seeds (sunflower, sesame, pumpkin), whole grains, organ meats	glands, heart, kidneys, nerves	cell oxidation & respiration, metabolism (protein, fat, sugar), glandular & nervous system stimulation	heart disease, nervous & glandular disorders	alcoholism, asthma, atherosclerosis, cholesterol (high), emphysema, heart disease, headaches, insomnia, poor circulation, premature aging, rheumatism, shortness of breath
C Ascorbic Acid Water Soluble Augmenting Nutrients: all vitamins & minerals, bioflavonoids, calcium, magnesium SR = 1–4 gm. to bowel tolerance when ill	citrus fruits, cantaloupe, green peppers broccoli (cooked): 1 cup = 135 mg. oranges: 1 med. = 100 mg. peppers (green): 1 med. = 120 mg. grapefruit: 1 med. = 100 mg. papaya (raw): 1 lg. = 225 mg. strawberries: 1 cup = 90 mg.	adrenal glands, blood, capillary walls, connective tissue (skin, ligaments, bones), gums, heart, teeth	bone & tooth formation, collagen production, digestion, iodine conservation, healing (burns & wounds), red blood cell formation (hemorrhaging prevention), shock & infection resistance (colds), vitamin protection (oxidation)	anemia, bleeding gums, capillary wall ruptures, bruise easily, dental cavities, low infection resistance (colds), nosebleeds, poor digestion	alcoholism, allergies, atherosclerosis, arthritis, baldness, cholesterol (high), colds, cystitis, hypoglycemia, heart disease, hepatitis, insect bites, overweight, prickly heat, sinusitis, stress, tooth decay

Vitamin	Source	Body Parts Affected	Bodily Functions Facilitated	Deficiency Symptoms	Therapeutic Indications
D Calciferol Fat Soluble Augmenting Nutrients: A, choline, C, calcium, phosphorus SR = 50–500 IU	egg yolks, organ meats, bone meal, sunlight liver (beef): ¼ lb. = 40 IU milk: 1 cup = 100 IU salmon/tuna (canned): ¼ lb. = 300 IU	bones, heart, nerves, skin, teeth, thyroid gland	calcium & phosphorus metabolism (bone formation), heart action, nervous system maintenance, normal blood clotting, skin respiration	burning sensation (mouth & throat) diarrhea, insomnia, myopia, nervousness, poor metabolism, softening bones & teeth	acne, alcoholism, allergies, arthritis, cystitis, eczema, psoriasis, stress
E Tocopherol Fat Soluble Augmenting Nutrients: A, B complex, B₁, inositol, C, manganese, selenium,	dark green vegetables, eggs, liver, organ meats, wheat germ, vegetable oils, desiccated liver oatmeal (cooked): 1 cup = 7 IU	blood vessels, heart, lungs, nerves, pituitary gland, skin	aging retardation, anticlotting factor, blood cholesterol reduction, blood flow to heart, capillary wall strengthening, male fertility,	dry, dull or falling hair, enlarged prostate gland, gastrointestinal disease, heart disease, impotency, miscarriages,	allergies, arthritis, atherosclerosis, baldness, cholesterol (high), crossed eyes, cystitis, diabetes, heart disease (coronary thrombosis, angina

202

phosphorus SR = 100–1,200 IU	safflower oil: 1 tbsp. = 20 IU vegetable oils: 1 tbsp. = 12 IU peanuts (roasted with skin): 1 cup = 13 IU tomatoes: 2 med. = 3 IU wheat germ oil: 1 tbsp. = 40 IU	potency, lung protection (antipollution), muscle & nerve maintenance	muscular wasting, sterility	pectoris, rheumatic heart disease), menstrual problems, menopause, migraine headaches, myopia, overweight, phlebitis, sinusitis, stress, thrombosis, varicose veins. External: burns, scars, warts, wrinkles, wounds

Table 2

Minerals and Their Uses

Mineral	Source	Body Parts Affected	Bodily Functions Facilitated	Deficiency Symptoms	Therapeutic Indications
Calcium Augmenting Nutrients: A, C, D, F, iron, magnesium, manganese, phosphorus SR = 800–2,000 mg.	milk, cheese, molasses, yogurt, bone meal, dolomite almonds: 1 cup = 325 mg. American cheese: 1 slice = 200 mg. liver (beef): ¼ lb. = 500 mg.	blood, bones, heart, skin, soft tissue, teeth	bone/tooth formation, blood clotting, heart rhythm, nerve tranquilization, nerve transmission, muscle growth & contraction	heart palpitations, insomnia, muscle cramps, nervousness, arm & leg numbness, tooth decay	arthritis, aging symptoms (backache, bone pain, finger tremors), foot/leg cramps, insomnia, menstrual cramps, menopause problems, nervousness, overweight, premenstrual tension, rheumatism

Nutrient	Sources	Body Parts	Function	Deficiency Symptoms	Excess Symptoms
Chromium SR = 100–1,000 mcg.	brewer's yeast, clams, corn oil, whole grain cereals	blood, circulatory system	blood sugar level, glucose metabolism (energy)	atherosclerosis, glucose intolerance in diabetics	diabetes, hypoglycemia
Copper Augmenting Nutrients: cobalt, iron, zinc SR = 2–5 mg.	legumes, nuts, organ meats, seafood, raisins, molasses, bone meal Brazil nuts: 1 cup = 4 mg. soybeans: 1 cup = 2 mg.	blood, bones, circulatory system, hair, skin	bone formation, hair & skin color, healing processes of body, hemoglobin & red blood cell formation	general weakness, impaired respiration, skin sores	anemia, baldness
Iodine SR = not established	seafood, kelp tablets, salt (iodized)	hair, nails, skin, teeth, thyroid gland	energy production, metabolism (excess fat), physical & mental development	cold hands & feet, dry hair, irritability, nervousness, obesity	atherosclerosis, hair problems, goiter, hyperthyroidism

Mineral	Source	Body Parts Affected	Bodily Functions Facilitated	Deficiency Symptoms	Therapeutic Indications
Iron Augmenting Nutrients: B₁₂, folic acid, C, calcium, cobalt, copper, phosphorus SR = 15–50 mg.	blackstrap molasses, eggs, fish, organ meats, poultry, wheat germ, desiccated liver liver (beef): ¼ lb. = 200 mg. shredded wheat: 1 biscuit = 30 mg.	blood, bones, nails, skin, teeth	hemoglobin production, stress & disease resistance	breathing difficulties, brittle nails, iron deficiency anemia (pale skin, fatigue), constipation	alcoholism, anemia, colitis, menstrual problems
Magnesium Augmenting Nutrients: B₆, C, D, calcium, phosphorus SR = 300–500 mg.	bran, honey, green vegetables, nuts, seafood, spinach, bone meal, kelp tablets bran flakes: 1 cup = 90 mg. peanuts (roasted with skin):	arteries, bones, heart, muscles, nerves, teeth	acid/alkaline balance, blood sugar metabolism (energy), metabolism (calcium & vitamin C)	confusion, disorientation, easily aroused anger, nervousness, rapid pulse, tremors	alcoholism, cholesterol (high), depression, heart conditions, kidney stones, nervousness, prostate troubles, sensitivity to noise, stomach

Mineral	Food Sources	Body Location	Functions	Deficiency Symptoms	Excess Symptoms
	1 cup = 420 mg. tuna fish (canned): ½ lb. = 150 mg.				acidity, tooth decay, overweight
Manganese SR = 5–50 mg.	bananas, bran, celery, cereals, egg yolks, green leafy vegetables, legumes, liver, nuts, pineapples, whole grains	brain, mammary glands, muscles, nerves	enzyme activation, reproduction & growth, hormone production, tissue respiration, vitamin B_1 metabolism, vitamin E utilization	ataxia (muscle coordination failure), dizziness, ear noises, loss of hearing	allergies, asthma, diabetes, fatigue
Phosphorus Augmenting Nutrients: A, D, F, calcium, iron, manganese SR = 800–1,000 mg.	eggs, fish, grains, glandular meats, meat, poultry, yellow cheese calf liver: ¼ lb. = 600 mg. milk/yogurt: 1 cup = 230 mg. eggs (cooked): 1 med. = 110 mg.	bones, brain, nerves, teeth	bone/tooth formation, cell growth & repair, energy production, heart muscle contraction, kidney function, metabolism (calcium, sugar), nerve & muscle activity, vitamin utilization	appetite loss, fatigue, irregular breathing, nervous disorders, overweight, weight loss	arthritis, stunted growth in children, stress, tooth & gum disorders

Mineral	Source	Body Parts Affected	Bodily Functions Facilitated	Deficiency Symptoms	Therapeutic Indications
Potassium Augmenting Nutrients: Vitamin B₆, sodium SR = 500 mg. several gm.	dates, figs, peaches, tomato juice, blackstrap molasses, peanuts, raisins, seafood apricots (dried): 1 cup = 1,450 mg. bananas: 1 med. = 500 mg. flounder (baked): ¼ lb. = 650 mg. potatoes (baked): 1 med. = 500 mg. sunflower seeds: 1 cup = 900 mg.	blood, heart, kidneys, muscles, nerves, skin	heartbeat, rapid growth, muscle contraction, nerve tranquilization	acne, continuous thirst, dry skin, constipation, general weakness, insomnia, muscle damage, nervousness, slow irregular heartbeat, weak reflexes	acne, alcoholism, allergies, burns, colic in infants, diabetes, high blood pressure, heart disease (angina pectoris, congestive heart failure, myocardial infarction)

Selenium SR = 10–100 mcg.	whole grains, garlic, asparagus, fish	cell membrane	resistance to cancer, heart disease, cell membrane integrity, heavy metal poisoning	muscle wasting, blood hemolytic problems, aging blood pigment, pancreatic insufficiency	heavy metal toxicity, cancer, heart disease, muscular diseases
Sodium Augmenting Nutrients: Vitamin D, potassium SR = 100–500 mg.	salt, milk, cheese, seafood	blood, lymph system, muscles, nerves	normal cellular fluid level, proper muscle contraction	appetite loss, intestinal gas, muscle shrinkage, vomiting, weight loss	dehydration, fever, heat stroke
Sulfur Augmenting Nutrients: B complex, B₁, biotin, pantothenic acid SR = not established	bran, cheese, clams, eggs, nuts, fish, wheat germ	hair, nails, nerves, skin	collagen synthesis, body tissue formation	not known	arthritis External: skin disorders (eczema, dermatitis, psoriasis)

Mineral	Source	Body Parts Affected	Bodily Functions Facilitated	Deficiency Symptoms	Therapeutic Indications
Zinc Augmenting Nutrients: A (high intake), calcium, copper, phosphorus SR = 15–50 mg.	brewer's yeast, liver, seafood, soybeans, spinach, sunflower seeds, mushrooms	blood, heart, prostate gland	burn & wound healing, carbohydrate digestion, prostate gland function, reproductive organ growth & development, sex organ growth & maturity, vitamin B₁, phosphorus & protein metabolism	delayed sexual maturity, fatigue, loss of taste, poor appetite, prolonged wound healing, retarded growth, sterility	alcoholism, atherosclerosis, baldness, cirrhosis, diabetes, internal & external wound & injury healing, high cholesterol (eliminates deposits), infertility

This table is not intended to be used for diagnostic or prescriptive purposes. For any treatment or diagnosis of illness, please see your physician. The use of certain dietary supplements may result in allergic reactions in some individuals; consult your physician.

AFTERWORD

I grew up under the shadow of the mushroom cloud. What difference did it make if I took sugar in my coffee or relished the fat on my steak?

Seeing my relatives living long lives, I never doubted the indestructibility of my body—at least by disease. On some vague principle that we have mental control over our health, I never involved myself with doctors or medicine, once I had escaped from the routine antibiotics of youth.

As a writer and researcher in the health field, I developed a broad familiarity with orthodox and unorthodox approaches to wellness. But never being seriously ill myself, I never felt compelled to apply this knowledge in my own life.

Suddenly, I had arrived at the brink of middle age. By coincidence I happened to be working on two books about aging. What ensued might be called a midlife meta-health crisis. Although I was fitter than I had been in my reckless youth, I now had to consider the possibility that doing *nothing* would no longer be enough.

I was already familiar with all the advice about diet and vitamin and mineral supplements. But if I were to follow all this advice, I would be carrying around a suit-case full of pills. How was I to sort it all out?

In the course of working on this book, the path has

become clearer. Looking at my family's history of possibly hereditary diseases, at the dietary and life-style stresses to which I had been subjected over a lifetime of heedlessness, I discovered a pattern—a few supplements and a set of simple dietary guidelines. Over and over again, the same nutritional strategies would apply to me in the various preventive packages that Michael Weiner and I were developing in this book.

Hopefully, our recommendations will come together for you in as clear a pattern. For each person it will be a little different; but underlying the specific recommendations there is an *attitude* that can make a big difference in the way we age. That attitude can be summed up in the following precepts:

1. A *major* goal as we age should be to maintain good health.

2. The diseases of middle and old age are largely *preventable*.

3. To prevent these diseases, we must become our *own* "doctors," thoughtfully laying a dietary groundwork for long-range health.

4. Not only must we correct our own bad dietary habits, but we must also *confront* the massive medicine and food industries, and learn to resist their seductive marketing techniques.

5. Taking such a stand *may* be a little less convenient, a little more expensive, and a little less "fun" than the way we have been accustomed to eating; but it gives us greater control over our lives. And it produces *noticeable* results!

Our planet is reaching the limits of the demands we can make upon it. Just as we must learn to conserve our precious energy resources and draw upon the free energy in nature, so must we learn to derive maximum benefits from our finite food supply.

Living in a nation of abundance, we use food for recreation rather than simple nourishment. The nutrients we waste, destroy, and overconsume each day might sustain the life of a less fortunate sister or brother in some far part of the globe.

Eating wisely is also eating with *respect*—respect for our own bodies; respect for our fellow humans with whom we share earth's bounty; and respect for the planet itself.

May all three endure in health!

San Francisco, 1982   KATHLEEN GOSS

APPENDIX

Table A.1

Vitamin A-Rich Foods

Food	Serving Size	IU per Serving
Beef liver	2 slices, pan fried	40,050
Carrots, dark orange	⅔ cup, cooked	10,500
Sweet potatoes	1 baked, medium size	8,910
Green leafy vegetables	½ cup, cooked	7,870
Cantaloupes	½ melon	6,800
Dried apricots	½ cup, cooked	4,200
Pumpkins	½ cup, cooked	3,840
Squash, winter	½ cup, boiled	3,500
Broccoli	⅔ cup, cooked	2,500
Tomatoes	1 medium	1,350
Fresh fruits (apricots, nectarines, peaches, cherries, watermelon, etc.)		100–2,700
Lettuce	4–5 small leaves	950
Asparagus	6 stalks	900
Milk (whole)	1 pint	740
Eggs	1 average size	590
Ice cream	⅙ quart	520
Cream cheese	1 ounce	460
Butter	1 pat	330

Source: Briggs and Calloway, *Nutrition and Physical Fitness.*

Table A.2

*Choline-Rich Foods**

egg yolks
whole grains
legumes (soybeans, peas, & beans)
meats
wheat germ

---

*Exact values are not available.

Table A.3

Magnesium Content in Sample Foods

Food	mg./100 gm.
Coffee, instant (dry powder)	456
Cocoa, dry powder	420
Wheat bran	420
Wheat germ	336
Soybeans	265
Yeast, brewer's	231
Walnuts, black	190
Peanuts, roasted	173
Flour, whole wheat	133
Beet greens*	106
Spinach*	88
Swiss chard*	65
Turnip greens*	58
Cheddar cheese	45
Peas	35
Bread, white	22
Rice, white	8

*Boiling vegetables removes the magnesium, so *save the water* for gravies, soups, etc.

Table A.4

*Zinc-Rich Foods**

Oysters
Clams
Shellfish
Seafood
Muscle meats
Whole grains
Wheat germ
Legumes
Nuts & seeds (especially pumpkin
    & sunflower seeds)
Eggs

---

* Exact values are omitted, but be aware that zinc is *low* in vegetables, fruits, and refined foods. The zinc found in *animal* foods is absorbed more readily than from plant foods and *vegetarians* must be sure they get enough zinc. Needs for alcohol drinkers, pregnant women, and those taking steroids (birth control pills) are greatly increased.

REFERENCES

Alvares, Olav. "Vitamin C and Periodontal Disease." *Journal of the American Medical Association*, August 14, 1981.

Ames, Bruce; Cathcart, Richard; Schwiers, Elizabeth; and Hochstein, Paul. "Uric Acid Provides an Antioxidant Defense in Humans Against Oxidant- and Radical-Caused Aging and Cancer: A Hypothesis." *Proceedings of the National Academy of Science*, 1981, 78(11):6858–62.

Anderson, James. "Fiber, Carbohydrate, and Diabetes." *Nutrition and the M.D.*, 1981, 6(7):1–2.

Arthritis Foundation. *Arthritis and Nutrition*. Atlanta, Georgia, 1980.

———. *Arthritis: The Basic Facts*. Atlanta, Georgia, 1978.

Baraona, Enrique, and Lieber, Charles S. "Effects of Ethanol on Lipid Metabolism." *Journal of Lipid Research*, 1979, 20:289–306.

Barton-Wright, E. C., and Elliott, W. A. "The Pantothenic Acid Metabolism of Rheumatoid Arthritis." *Lancet*, October 26, 1963.

Bingham, Robert. "Nutrition in the Treatment of Arthritis." *Journal of Applied Nutrition*, 1972, 25:112–25.

———, Bellew, Bernard A.; and Bellew, Joeva G. "Yucca Plant Saponin in the Management of Arthritis." *Journal of Applied Nutrition*, 1972, :45–51.

Bordia, Arun. "Effect of Garlic on Blood Lipids in Patients with Coronary Heart Disease." *American Journal of Clinical Nutrition*, 1981, 34:2100–03.

Burkitt, Denis P. "Some Neglected Leads to Cancer Causation." *Journal of the National Cancer Institute*, 1971, 47(4):913–19.

Butler, Robert N. *Why Survive?* New York: Harper & Row, Publishers, 1975.

Caster, W. O. "The Role of Nutrition in Human Aging." In Morris Rockstein and Marvin L. Sussman, eds., *Nutrition, Longevity, and Aging*. New York: Academic Press, Inc., 1976.

Cheraskin, E., Ringsdorf, W. M., and Clark, J. W. *Diet and Disease*. New Canaan, Conn.: Keats Publishing Co., 1968.

———, and Ringsdorf, W. M. *Psychodietetics*. New York: Bantam, 1976.

Cherkin, Arthur. "Higher Cognitive Processes." In Gabe J. Maletta, ed., *Survey Report on the Aging Nervous System*. Bethesda, Md.: U.S. Dept. of Health, Education and Welfare, Public Health Service, National Institutes of Health, 1975.

Cleave, T. L. "The Neglect of Natural Principles in Current Medical Practice. *Journal of the Royal Naval Medical Service*, 1956, 42:55–83.

Daniell, Harry W. "Smoker's Wrinkles: A Study in the Epidemiology of 'Crow's Feet.' " *Annals of Internal Medicine*, 1971, 75:873–80.

Davis, Adelle. *Let's Eat Right to Keep Fit*. New York: Signet, 1970.

Diamond, Marian Cleeves. "The Aging Brain: Some Enlightening and Optimistic Results. *American Scientist*, 1978, 66:66–71.

Doll, Richard, and Peto, Richard. "The Causes of Cancer: Quantitative Estimates of Avoidable Risks of Cancer in the United States Today." *Journal of the National Cancer Institute*, 1981, 66(6):1191–1308.

Fair, William R. *Medical World News*, February 7, 1977:57.

Fellman, Bruce. "A Nutritional Plan for Terrific Teeth." *Prevention*, December 1981:59–63.

Fredericks, Carlton. *Breast Cancer: A Nutritional Approach*. New York: Grosset & Dunlap, Inc., 1977.

———. *Low Blood Sugar and You*. New York: Grosset & Dunlap, Inc., 1969.

Friedman, Gerald. "Diet in the Treatment of Diabetes Mellitus." In R. S. Goodhart and Maurice E. Shils, eds., *Modern Nutrition in Health and Disease*. Philadelphia: Lea & Febiger, 1980.

Gerritson, George C. "The Role of Nutrition to Diabetics in Relation to Age. In Morris Rockstein and Marvin L. Sussman, eds., *Nutrition, Longevity and Aging*. New York: Academic Press, Inc., 1976.

Goldberg, R.; Szklo, M.; Tonascia, J. A.; and Kennedy, H. L. "Time Trends in Prognosis of Patients with Myocardial Infarction: A Population-Based Study." *Johns Hopkins Medical Journal*, 1979, 144:73–80.

Graham, S.; Dayal, H.; Swanson, M. et al. "Diet in the Epidemiology of Cancer of the Colon and Rectum." *Journal of the National Cancer Institute*, 1978, 61:709–14.

———, and Mettlin, C. "Diet and Colon Cancer." *American Journal of Epidemiology*, 1979, 109:1–26.

Gruberg, Edward R., and Raymond, Stephen A. "Beyond Cholesterol: A New Theory of Arteriosclerosis." *Atlantic Monthly*, May 1979:59–65.

Guggenheim, Y. K. "Forerunners of the Vitamin Doctrine." *Korof (Bulletin of the History of Medical Science)*, 1979, 7:181–94.

Haenszel, W.; Locke, F. B.; and Segi, M. "A Case-Control Study of Large Bowel Cancer in Japan." *Journal of the National Cancer Institute*, 1980, 64:17–22.

Harris, Seale. *Journal of the American Medical Association*, 1924, 83:729.

Henig, Robin Marantz. *The Myth of Senility*. Garden City, N.Y.: Anchor Press/Doubleday, 1981.

Hoffer, Abram, and Walker, Morton. *Nutrients to Age Without Senility*. New Canaan, Conn.: Keats Publishing Co., 1980.

Johnson, Francois C. "Carcinogenesis, Vascular Disease, and the Free Radical Reaction." *Nutrition and Cancer*, 1982, 3(3):117–121.

Jones, Irving. "The Skin: Mirror of Health." *Life and Health*, March 1976:9.

Kark, J. D.; Smith, A. H.; Switzer, B. R.; and Hames, C. G. "Serum Vitamin A (Retinol) and Cancer Incidence in Evans County, Georgia." *Journal of the National Cancer Institute*, 1981, 66:7–16.

Kaufman, William. *The Common Form of Joint Dysfunction: Its Incidence and Treatment*. Brattleboro, Vt.: Hildreth, 1949.

Kinderlehrer, Jane. "B$_6$—Maybe the Answer to Heart Disease." *Prevention*, September 1979, 138–45.

Klatsky, Arthur L.; Friedman, Gary D.; and Siegelaub, Abraham D. "Alcohol Consumption Before Myocardial Infarction: Results from the Kaiser Permanente Epidemiologic Study of Myocardial Infarction." *Annals of Internal Medicine*, 1974, 81:294–301.

Kolodzey, Judy. "Best Foods for Healthy Hair." *Prevention*, May 1981:101–06.

Kornecki, Elizabeth, and Feinberg, Harold. *American Journal of Physiology*, 1980, 238(1).

Kuhn, Maggie. "Interview with Maggie Kuhn." *New Age*, February 1979.

Kunin, Richard. *Mega-Nutrition*. New York: McGraw-Hill Book Company, 1980.

Lages, William L. *Living it up with Arthritis: Diet and Arthritis*. San Francisco: Arthritis Foundation.

Lasker, Gabriel W., and Kaplan, Bernice. "Graying of the Hair and Mortality." *Social Biology*, 1975, 21(3):290–95.

Levy, Robert I. "Declining Mortality in Coronary Heart Disease." *Arteriosclerosis*, 1981, 1(5):312–25.

Lubowe, Irwin. "Treatment of the Aging Skin by Dermatologic Methods." *Journal of the American Geriatrics Society*, 1976, 24(1):25–28.

Mann, John A. *Secrets of Life Extension*. Berkeley: And/Or Press, Inc., 1980.

Mazer, Eileen. "The Exciting News about Vitamin B$_6$." *Prevention*, January 1982:18–26.

McGill, Henry C., Jr.; McMahan, Alex; and Wene, Jamie Dollahite. "Unresolved Problems in the Diet-Heart Issue." *Arteriosclerosis*, 1981, 1:164–76.

National Heart, Lung, and Blood Institute. "The NHLBI Consensus Development Conference Statement on Coronary Artery Bypass Surgery; Scientific and Clinical Aspects." *New England Journal of Medicine*, 1981, 304:680–84.

Nutrition Reviews. "Alcohol Consumption and High-Density Lipoprotein Cholesterol in Marathon Runners." August 1981, 39(8).

Padus, Amrika. "Yes! You Can Prevent Wrinkles!" *Prevention*, November 1981:57–62.

Pathak, M. A.; Fitzpatrick, T. B.; and Frenk, E. "Evaluation of Topical Agents that Prevent Sunburn—Superiority of Para-Aminobenzoic Acid and its Ester in Ethyl Alcohol. *New England Journal of Medicine*, 1968, 280(26):1459–63.

Peterson, L. N. "Nutritional Influence on Periodontal Disease." *Journal of Applied Nutrition*, 1972, 24:87–105.

Pfeiffer, Carl C. *Mental and Elemental Nutrients*. New Canaan, Conn.: Keats Publishing Co., 1975.

Phillips, Nancy R.; Havel, Richard J.; and Kane, John P. "Levels and Interrelationships of Serum and Lipoprotein Cholesterol and Triglycerides; Association with Adiposity and the Consumption of Ethanol, Tobacco and Beverages Containing Caffeine." *Arteriosclerosis*, 1981, 1:13–24.

Price, Weston A. *Nutrition and Physical Degeneration, Isolated and Modernized Peoples*. Santa Monica: Price-Pottenger Foundation, 1970.

Rawson, Rulon W. "The Role of Nutrition in the Etiology and Prevention of Cancer." *Nutrition and Cancer*, 1980, 2(1):17–21.

Reuben, David. *The Save Your Life Diet*. New York: Ballantine, 1975.

Robertson, Laurel; Flinders, Carol; and Godfrey, Bronwen. *Laurel's Kitchen*. New York: Bantam, 1978.

Rudel, Lawrence; Leathers, Charles W.; Bond, M. Gene; and Bullock, Bill C. "Dietary Ethanol-Induced Modifications in Hyperlipoproteinemia and Atherosclerosis in Non-Human Primates *(Macaca nemestrina)*." *Arteriosclerosis*, 1981, 1(2).

Ruffer, M. A. "On Arterial Lesions Found in Egyptian Mummies." *Journal of Pathology and Bacteriology*, 1911, 15:453.

Sandler, Rivka Black, and Herbert, David L. "Quantitative Bone Assessments: Applications and Expectations." *Journal of the American Geriatrics Society*, 1981, 24(3):97.

Selden, Gary. *Aphrodisia*. New York: E. P. Dutton & Co., Inc., 1979.

Sheehy, Gail. *Passages*. New York: Bantam, 1977.

Shubik, Philippe H. "Food Additives, Contaminants, and Cancer." *Preventive Medicine*, 1980, 9:197–201.

Sieve, B. F. "Clinical Achromotrichia." *Science*, 1941, 94:257.

Starr, Barnard D., and Weiner, Marcella Bakur. *The Starr-Weiner Report on Sex and Sexuality in the Mature Years*. New York: Stein and Day Publishers, 1981.

Steason, William B.; Neff, Raymond K.; Miettinen, Ollis; and Jick, Hershel. "Alcohol Consumption and Nonfatal Myocardial Infarction." *American Journal of Epidemiology*, 1976, 104(6):603–7.

Taylor, C. B. et al. "Spontaneously Occurring Angiotoxic Derivatives of Cholesterol." *American Journal of Clinical Nutrition*, 1979, 32:40–57.

Time. "Building up Brittle Bones." December 7, 1981:100.

Wald, N.; Idle, M.; Boreham, J. et al. "Low Serum-Vitamin-A and Subsequent Risk of Cancer." *Lancet*, 1980, 2:813–18.

Weaver, Arthur; Fleming, Susan M.; and Smith, Donald B. "Mouthwash and Oral Cancer: Carcinogen or Coincidence?" *Journal of Oral Surgery*, 1979, 37:250–53.

Weiner, Michael, and Rothschild, Jonathan. "The Vitamin that Likes Oxygen." *Runner's World*, February 1980:87–89.

————. *The Way of the Skeptical Nutritionist*. New York: Macmillan Publishing Co., Inc., 1981.

Williams, Roger J. *Nutrition Against Disease*. New York: Bantam, 1981.

————. *The Prevention of Alcoholism Through Nutrition*. New York: Bantam, 1981.

Yates, John. "B_6 and A–1 Circulation." *Prevention*, July 1980:56–59.

Zarafonetis, C.J.D. "Darkening of Gray Hair During Paraamino-Benzoic Acid Therapy." *Journal of Investigative Dermatology*, 1960, 15:398–401.

INDEX

ABOUT THE AUTHORS

MICHAEL WEINER holds a Ph.D. from the University of California, Berkeley in Nutritional Ethnomedicine. He is the author of *Weiner's Herbal* and *Earth Medicine-Earth Foods* which has over 150,000 copies in print. His latest book published by Bantam is entitled *The Complete Book of Homeopathy*. He is on the faculty of the University of Santa Cruz and is Visiting Scholar at the Hebrew University School of Pharmacy.

KATHLEEN GOSS is a writer, researcher, and editor who is committed to the ongoing revolution in health and consciousness, and who uses her scholarly skills to interpret nonorthodox points of view for a popular audience. With Dr. Weiner she has also co-authored *The Art of Feeding Children Well* and *The Complete Book of Homeopathy*. She lives in San Francisco.

How's Your Health?

Bantam publishes a line of informative books, written by top experts to help you toward a healthier and happier life.

NEED MORE INFORMATION ON YOUR HEALTH AND NUTRITION?

Read the books that will lead you to
a happier and healthier life.

We Deliver!
And So Do These Bestsellers.

☐	23714	**THE DEVIL IN CONNECTICUT** by G. Brittle	$3.50
☐	22634	**THE AMITYVILLE HORROR** by Jay Anson	$3.50
☐	23695	**TOUGH LOVE** by P. & D. York w/ T. Wachtel	$3.50
☐	05042	**HEARTS WE BROKE LONG AGO** by M. Shain (A Large Format Book)	$10.95
☐	22646	**SOME MEN ARE MORE THAN PERFECT** by Merle Shain	$2.95
☐	22649	**WHEN LOVERS ARE FRIENDS** by Merle Shain	$2.95
☐	05035	**OUT ON A LIMB** by Shirley MacLaine (A Hardcover Book)	$14.95
☐	01457	**YOUR ACHING BACK** by A. A. White III, M.D. (A Hardcover Book)	$7.95
☐	23029	**HAVING IT BOTH WAYS** by E. Denholtz	$3.50
☐	23568	**GET A JOB IN 60 SECONDS** by Steve Kravette	$2.95
☐	23355	**'LUDES** by Benjamin Stein	$3.50
☐	22616	**THE DEMON SYNDROME** by Nancy Osborn Ishmael	$2.95
☐	23563	**THE ONLY INVESTMENT GUIDE YOU'LL EVER NEED** by Andrew Tobias	$3.95
☐	23188	**BEVERLY HILLS DIET LIFETIME PLAN** by Judy Mazel	$3.95
☐	22661	**UP THE FAMILY TREE** by Teresa Bloomingdale	$2.95
☐	22701	**I SHOULD HAVE SEEN IT COMING WHEN THE** **RABBIT DIED** by Teresa Bloomingdale	$2.75
☐	22576	**PATHFINDERS** by Gail Sheehy	$4.50
☐	22585	**THE MINDS OF BILLY MILLIGAN** by Daniel Keyes	$3.95
☐	22771	**THE GREATEST SUCCESS IN THE WORLD** by Og Mandino	$2.75
☐	23271	**WHY DO I THINK I'M NOTHING WITHOUT A MAN?** by Dr. P. Russianoff	$3.50
☐	23296	**BH&G STEP-BY-STEP HOUSEHOLD REPAIRS** by BH&G Editors	$3.50
☐	20621	**THE PILL BOOK** by Dr. Gilbert Simon & Dr. Harold Silverman	$3.95
☐	23111	**GUINNESS BOOK OF WORLD RECORDS—21st ed.** by McWhirter	$3.95